D1546302

AUTHORS

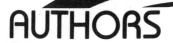

GAIL WALRAVEN
Chief, Education and Training
Office of Emergency Medical Services
San Diego, California

JOSIE HARDING R.N.
Instructor, EMS Training Program
San Diego, California

KAREN MILAZZO LeBLANC R.N.
Instructor, EMS Training Program
San Diego, California

GINGER MURPHY R.N., B.S.N.
Instructor, EMS Training Program
San Diego, California

MARGARET F. NERNEY R.N., B.S.N.
Instructor, EMS Training Program
San Diego, California

Manual of

ADVANCED PREHOSPITAL CARE

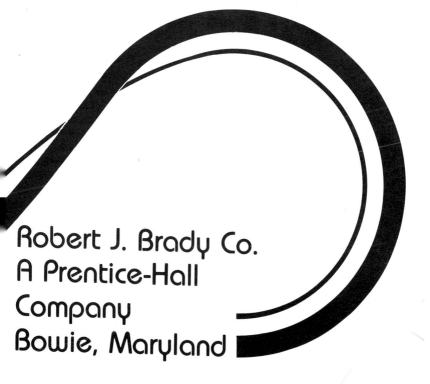

Robert J. Brady Co.
A Prentice-Hall
Company
Bowie, Maryland

Executive Editor	Richard A. Weimer
Production Editor	Charlett Bundy
Art Director	Don Sellers
Text/Cover Design	Laura Lammens

Manual of Advanced Prehospital Care

Library of Congress Cataloging in Publication Data

Main entry under title:

Manual of advanced prehospital care.

Includes index.
1. Medical emergencies. I. Walraven, Gail, 1949– [DNLM: 1. Emergency health services—Handbooks. 2. Allied health personnel—Handbooks. WX215 M294]

RC86.7.M35   616'.025   78-57615
ISBN 0-87618-995-8

Prentice-Hall International, Inc., London
Prentice-Hall of Australia, Pty., Ltd., Sydney
Prentice-Hall of India Private Limited, New Delhi
Prentice-Hall of Japan, Inc., Tokyo
Prentice-Hall of Southeast Asia Pte. Ltd., Singapore
Whitehall Books, Limited, Wellington, New Zealand
Printed in the United States of America

79 80 81 82   10 9 8 7 6 5 4 3 2

CONTENTS

FOREWORD

Emergency medical care has become a national health care priority at all governmental and professional levels. This focus on improving the care of emergency patients is the result of the recognition of the enormous toll of death and disability arising from emergency medical conditions. For example:

- Each year in the United States, 115,000 people die of accidental injury—the largest cause of death in people under 45 years of age. Over 400,000 people per year are permanently disabled.*

- Over 1 million people die each year from heart attacks, half of those die before reaching medical help.*

- Seventy-five thousand severe burn injuries occur each year. Less than 7500 receive care by burn specialists in burn centers.

- Ten thousand spinal cord injuries occur each year, resulting in a lifetime of disability at great cost to our nation. Less than 1000 are cared for in specialized care centers.

- Five thousand additional deaths occur as a result of the myriad of other emergency medical conditions which strike us all.

It is not only the enormity of these figures that demands a solution, but also the fact that most of them are preventable with existing medical technology. The challenge of medicine today is to bring that technology to the patient in the prehospital setting within the necessary time frame. This is best accomplished by utilizing paramedics effectively and by delivering critically ill or injured patients to designated critical care centers for definitive care.

In recent years a segment of this total EMS system, prehospital care, has received great attention. Many pioneering programs across the country have shown the value and practicality of bringing

---

* These two emergency conditions alone account for approximately half of *all* death and disability in our country.

resuscitative emergency medical care to the patient in the field. They have shown that the physician and his back-up hospital resources can be brought to the scene, via the paramedic, to save lives. Many training programs have been developed to meet the needs of communities desiring to improve the prehospital care provided to their citizens.

In San Diego, where a comprehensive EMS system was also being developed, the training program took on a new dimension in medical education. For the first time, training focused on how to meet a medical system's manpower needs in number and function. Under the leadership of Gail Walraven, the authors of the *Manual of Advanced Prehospital Care* developed a model training program, first defining the role of the paramedic and those of the nurse and physician with whom he must work as a team member. Second, they identified the functions each must perform in providing prehospital medical care.

In order to best utilize these functions, instructional objectives (competencies) were developed along with evaluation criteria for both students and the training program. Maintenance of competencies through continuing education and evaluation was considered an integral part of the training program.

This book, *Manual of Advanced Prehospital Care,* is a reflection of this systems approach to the training of prehospital personnel, and is a major contribution to the advancement of *appropriate* prehospital care. It includes only what the paramedic must know in order to perform competently, omitting irrelevant material and any procedures which may only delay appropriate care in another phase of the system. It is equally applicable to all members of the prehospital team (physicians, nurses, and paramedics) since care appropriate to the scene is the common denominator of the book. The authors have extensive experience not only in training prehospital personnel, but also in field care, which contributes to the uniqueness and relevancy of the text. Although designed to meet the needs of paramedics in maintaining their competence, it will be of great assistance to existing training programs, both as part of their initial training efforts and as part of their competency maintenance and refresher training.

The sections on Treatment Protocols and Practical Skills, along with specific procedural guidelines and self-assessment questions, add a new dimension to the book which will be extremely valuable to paramedic instructors, EMS Systems Medical Directors, and paramedics themselves.

The authors are to be congratulated for this excellent contribution to the field of prehospital care. The *Manual of Advanced Prehospital*

Care should be part of every paramedic's library and part of every training program's teaching resource.

Sylvia Micik, M.D.,
Director,
Division of Emergency Medical Services,
Department of Public Health,
County of San Diego, California

PREFACE

During the past few years, medical professionals across the country have been working diligently to upgrade prehospital emergency medical care by offering more sophisticated training to the field providers. The attention now being given to this specialized area of patient care has created a need for more information to supplement training programs. Additionally, with recertification testing a reality, paramedics must accept the professional responsibility for maintaining their level of competence; however, in order for them to meet that responsibility, the necessary information must be made available in a practical efficient format. To that end we set about developing a comprehensive compilation of all the information considered essential to the safe and effective field performance of a paramedic.

The *Manual of Advanced Prehospital Care* is not a textbook; it is not designed to teach concepts or explain emergency care to those just entering the field. Rather, it is written for experienced paramedics who have already had basic instruction in these areas. The format is encyclopedic in that it highlights all major points without providing in-depth instruction or explanation of this information. The book is designed to serve as a reference source and self-evaluation guide. It contains self-assessment questions so that paramedics may test themselves to identify what they need to review further.

Although intended primarily to help the certified paramedic prepare for recertification, the text can also be of value to those who wish to use it concurrently with initial instruction. It helps the paramedic distinguish between "need to know" and "nice to know," — especially during the initial training course, when so much information is delivered so quickly that it becomes overwhelming. The *Manual of Advanced Prehospital Care* attempts to assist the paramedic in putting this wealth of information into perspective. It is ideal for studying either for recertification or for initial training exams.

The manual is organized into five major categories of independent medical knowledge. Section I, *Medical Management,* provides short narratives on each of 22 common medical and traumatic conditions including a brief pathophysiology, the clinical manifestations, and the field treatment for each. The second section is *Treatment Protocols,* which augments Section I by categorizing these clinical conditions according to a patient's presenting complaint. Each protocol includes a summary of patient assessment questions, differential diagnosis, field treatment, pediatric notes, and transport guidelines. Section III, *Pharmacology,* includes 33 drug and IV solution profiles, conversion tables, and information on 25 classifications of medications commonly found in the home. The fourth section, *Arrhythmias,* offers a brief discussion of electrophysiology and a concise summation of 23 basic arrhythmias. Also included are several EKG stumbling blocks and 60 practice situations for arrhythmia interpretation. The last section deals with *Practical Skills.* For each of the 25 skills presented there is a brief narrative that includes definitions, indications, contraindications, and special precautions. Following the narrative is an outline of the steps to be required for performing the skill.

The *Manual of Advanced Prehospital Care* is a simple, easy-to-read summary of all the knowledge, skills, and experience we could convey on paper. The format is easy to follow, with materials outlined clearly and concisely from the perspective of the field provider. We have omitted irrelevant topics and have made no attempt to discuss inhospital procedures. This is truly a *field manual,* written by people with extensive field experience, and with input from countless field providers.

San Diego, California

Gail Walraven
Josie Harding
Karen LeBlanc
Ginger Murphy
Margie Nerney

ACKNOWLEDGMENTS

No book can go to press without a list of accolades for all of the individuals who contributed their time, thoughts and expertise to its making. True to this tradition, we extend our most sincere appreciation to Sylvia Micik, M.D., Director of Emergency Medical Services, San Diego County, whose enthusiasm, support, and dedication to the public welfare produced the EMS system in which we were all able to grow. The patient assessment section was developed with inspiration from the writings of Ron Stewart, M.D., and from a working model developed by Firefighter-Paramedic Bob Blizzard, Lakeside Fire Department, California. Our special thanks go to both of them.

Most importantly, we appreciate and compliment the meticulous efforts expended by the following reviewers to strengthen and polish the original manuscript.

David Allan, M.D.
John Bachman, M.D.
David R. Boyd, M.D.C.M.
Karen Campbell, R.N.
Ellen Gavel, R.N.
Steve Karas, M.D.
Costas Lambrew, M.D.
Capt. F. C. Leisse, MC, USN
Kenneth L. Mattox, M.D.
Jeffery R. McDonald, M.D.
Charles Phillips, M.D.
Elaine Siner, R.N.
Stan Zydlow, M.D.

There is no way to give thanks to all of those along the way who molded our experiences, opened our minds, and shared in our discoveries, but we cannot close this narrative without acknowledging the support we received from our families and friends.

COMMON ABBREVIATIONS

Abbreviation	Meaning
$\bar{a}$	before
ABC	airway, breathing, circulation
ALS	advanced life support
AMI	acute myocardial infarction
amps	ampules
ANS	autonomic nervous systrem
ARP	absolute refractory period
ASA	aspirin
ASHD	arteriosclerotic heart disease
AT	atrial tachycardia
AV	atrioventricular
bicarb	sodium bicarbonate
BID	twice a day
BLS	basic life support
BP	blood pressure
BS	blood sugar
$\bar{c}$	with
Ca^+	calcium
$CaCl_2$	calcium chloride
CAD	coronary artery disease
CC	chief complaint
cc	cubic centimeter
CCU	coronary care unit
CHB	complete heart block
CHF	congestive heart failure
Cl^-	chloride
cm	centimeter
CNS	central nervous system
c/o	complains of
CO	carbon monoxide
CO_2	carbon dioxide
Code 3	respond as rapidly as possible, red light and siren
COPD	chronic obstructive pulmonary disease
CPR	cardiopulmonary resuscitation
CSF	cerebrospinal fluid
CSM	carotid sinus massage
CV	cardiovascular
CVA	cerebrovascular accident

Abbreviation	Meaning
D/C	discontinue
dig	digitalis
DOA	dead on arrival
DOE	dyspnea on exertion
DM	diabetes mellitus
D/W, D₅W, 5% D/W	5% dextrose in water
D₅₀W, 50% D/W	50% dextrose in water
Dx	diagnosis
EA, EOA	esophageal obturator airway
ED	emergency department
EKG, ECG	electrocardiogram
Epi	epinephrine
ER	emergency room
ET	endotracheal
ETOH	alcohol
fib	fibrillation
fl	fluid
fx	fracture
GI	gastrointestinal
gm	gram
gr	grain
gt(t)	drop(s)
h, hr	hour
HBD	has been drinking
hx	history
IC	intracardiac
ICU	intensive care unit
IM	intramuscular
IV	intravenous
K$^+$	potassium
Kg	kilogram
KO	keep open
KVO	keep vein open
L	liter
LBB	left bundle branch
LOC	level of consciousness
μgtt	microdrops
MCl₁	modified chest lead, V₁
MD	doctor
mEq	milliequivalents
mg	milligram

Abbreviation	Meaning
MI	myocardial infarction
MIC	mobile intensive care
MICN	mobile intensive care nurse
MICU	mobile intensive care unit
min	minute
ml	milliliter
mm	millimeter
mv	millivolt
MS	morphine sulfate
Na+	sodium
NaCl	sodium chloride
NaHCO₃	sodium bicarbonate
NG, N/G	nasogastric
nitro	nitroglycerine
NPO	nothing by mouth
NS	normal saline
NSR	normal sinus rhythm
NTG	nitroglycerine
O₂	oxygen
OB	obstetrics
OD	overdose
OPP	organophosphate poisoning
OR	operating room
P	pulse
p̄	after
PAC	premature atrial contraction
PAM	Protopam®
PAT	paroxysmal atrial tachycardia
PE	physical exam, pulmonary edema
pedi	pediatric
PERL	pupils equal, reactive to light
PJC	premature junctional contraction
PNC	premature nodal contraction
PND	paraxysmal nocturnal dyspnea
po	orally, by mouth
PRI	P-R interval of EKG
pr	per rectum
prn	whenever necessary, as needed
PVC	premature ventricular contraction
q̄	every
QID	four times a day
R	respirations

Abbreviation	Meaning
RBB	right bundle branch
RBC	red blood cell
RHD	rheumatic heart disease
RL	Ringer's Lactate
R/O	rule out
RN	registered nurse
RRP	relative refractory period
Rx	treatment
s̄	without
SA	sinoatrial
SC	subcutaneous
sec	second
SICU	surgical intensive care unit
SIDS	sudden infant death syndrome
SL	sublingual
SOB	shortness of breath
SPA	salt poor albumin
SQ	subcutaneous
STAT	immediately
s/s	signs/symptoms
SVT	supraventricular tachycardia
Sx	symptoms
TIA	transient ischemic attack
TID	three times a day
TKO	to keep open
u.	unit
VF	ventricular fibrillation
VS	vital signs
VT	ventricular tachycardia
WAP	wandering atrial pacemaker
WBC	white blood cell
w/s	watt/second setting
x	times
y/o	years old

MEDICAL
MANAGEMENT

INTRODUCTION

This section on Medical Management lists alphabetically virtually all of the acute medical conditions which the paramedic can expect to find in a prehospital setting. A short narrative discusses each of these conditions, including a brief pathophysiology as it relates to symptoms, the clinical picture of the emergency stage, and the field treatment required to stabilize the patient. As with the other sections of *Manual of Advanced Prehospital Care,* this section does not attempt to teach, but does gather summary information into a clear synopsis of pertinent material.

Throughout the book, and specifically in the Medical Management section, an attempt has been made to standardize field care and drug dosages in compliance with existing standards established by organizations such as the American Heart Association.

To use this section, first read the narratives as they exist. Then go back and modify each one if necessary to coincide with the teachings and policies of your local program. Check with your instructors, medical advisors, and other resources to be certain your changes are accurate. Once these modifications are complete, you can use the narratives as a basis for study. To assess your retention and understanding of the material, complete the self-assessment questions at the end of the section. In order to be effective, the self-assessment section should be completed without using notes or other aides. If you desire further study, refer to the bibliography at the end of the book.

ASSESSMENT

Assessment of the total patient situation is the most important function you must perform. Without a systematic and thorough approach to assessment, vital aspects of the patient's condition might be overlooked. The order of assessment will vary according to each situation, but must always follow an organized format. Assessment techniques develop with practice but are rarely easy in the beginning. With practice and attention to detail, you can develop these skills into your most valuable tools.

The information presented here is offered only as a sample organizational plan for all the information that must be remembered during patient assessment. It is vital that each paramedic develop his or her own organized approach, and use that approach *consistently* in dealing with patients in the field. For continuity, the entire assessment process should be completed by a single paramedic whenever possible.

The Primary Survey

Patient assessment is divided into *primary* and *secondary* surveys. The primary survey includes evaluation of the scene and initial assessment of the patient. First, conduct a quick assessment of the scene to determine such things as a) the mechanism of injury, b) the number of patients to be treated, c) the need for extrication, and d) environmental dangers. During the primary survey, identify life-threatening situations and institute corrective measures. Your foremost consideration in *all* patients is the status of the ABCs:

AIRWAY
- Is it patent?
- Does the patient need positioning or suctioning?
- Are the respirations noisy, gurgling, or labored?
- Does the patient need an artificial airway?
- Is the chest wall intact?

BREATHING
- Is the patient breathing spontaneously?
- What is the quality and depth of respiration?

- What is the frequency of respiration?
- Does the patient need ventilatory assistance or support?

CIRCULATION
- Is the pulse palpable?
- Does the circulation need to be supported?
- What is the quality of the pulse?
- What is the skin color?
- Is there any obvious bleeding?

Each of these basic assessments must be made, and any deficiencies corrected, before continuing with a more sophisticated evaluation. During your primary survey you should also be looking for clues such as medication bottles, syringes, drugs, or weapons. It may be helpful to request the assistance of auxiliary personnel to assist you in your survey of the scene; this also frees you for patient care.

After the ABCs have been assessed and necessary support given, you must quickly evaluate the patient and determine whether immediate transport is needed. There are circumstances which cannot be corrected by prehospital intervention because they require the sophisticated support available only within the hospital. These situations are generally those that require surgery, but can include any condition where prehospital intervention is not actively helping the patient. Examples of such conditions include ruptured aneurysm, major trauma to the head, chest, or abdomen, or multisystem trauma, *where the patient is not compensating or is deteriorating.* Also, if your system requires radio contact but your communications are disrupted, it is wise to transport the patient without delay, continuing assessment enroute.

The Secondary Survey

If the patient does not require immediate transport, move on to the secondary survey for a more detailed assessment. The secondary survey consists of a) further investigation of the chief complaint, b) assessment of vital signs, c) gathering of a pertinent medical history, and d) performance of a manipulative physical exam.

Investigating the Chief Complaint

If the patient is conscious, determine why you were called and ask questions pertinent to the chief complaint. Pursue this line of questioning until a clear picture can be painted for the base hospital. Avoid "tunnel vision" which can result from focusing on one problem before you have investigated other possibilities. The following questions should help you gather a specific medical history.

1. *What is the chief complaint?*

   - Why was help requested?
   - How does the patient describe the problem?
   - When did it start?
   - What caused it?
   - Has it ever happened before?
   - How severe is it?
   - Does anything make it better or worse?
   - Was there any trauma?

2. *Are there any associated problems?*

   - Are there any other signs, symptoms, or injuries?
   - Is the patient taking any medications?
   - Is the patient seeing a private physician?
   - What is the past medical history?
   - Does the patient have any allergies?

Gathering the Vital Signs

While obtaining a detailed history, begin to gather vital signs by palpating a pulse and assessing the quality of respirations. Other vital signs should be assessed as quickly as possible. Table 1.1 lists the factors to be determined and reported for each of the vital sign categories.

In an unconscious patient, your job will be more difficult and your approach will vary. You will need to concentrate more on assessment of respirations, pupil reaction, response to painful or vocal stimuli, and motor function. You may be able to elicit a pertinent medical history from bystanders. Vital signs are extremely important in this situation and should be obtained without delay.

Table 1.1. Assessing Vital Signs

Vital signs	Factors to check
Blood pressure	systolic/diastolic; bilateral equality
Pulse	rate, rhythm, quality
Respirations	rate, rhythm, effectiveness, patterns
Level of consciousness	response to stimuli (including voice, touch and pain); orientation; motor response
Skin	color, temperature, moisture
Lungs	rales, wheezes, decreased or absent breath sounds
Pupils	equality; reaction to light (inappropriate in a conscious patient without neurological manifestations)
EKG	arrhythmias (monitor all patients with chest pain, respiratory distress, overdose, coma, drowning, or questionable diagnosis)

Performing a Physical Examination

The data you gather from a physical examination should provide some clues to the patient's problem, as well as direct you to areas of further patient assessment. While obtaining the history and establishing the chief complaint, begin performing a rapid head-to-toe exam. A complete physical exam, with appropriate concentration on specific areas of complaint, can be done in less than 2 minutes. The four basic evaluative maneuvers commonly used to conduct a physical exam are as follows:

INSPECTION
- Look at the patient.
- Note patient's coloring, positioning, and anxiety level.
- Look for chest wall movement or unusual posturing.
- Note patient's position relative to the surroundings.

- Examine patient front and back for obvious areas of injury.
- Look for guarding or other protective maneuvers.
- Look for evidence of chronic or acute disorders.

AUSCULTATION

- Listen to the chest to evaluate respiratory sounds and heart rate. (It is not appropriate to perform sophisticated auscultation of heart or bowel sounds in the prehospital setting, as the findings will not alter field treatment and will only cause a delay in transport.)

PALPATION

- Gently run your hands down the patient's body, checking for bleeding, areas of tenderness or deformity, or loss of sensation.

- Gently press thoracic cage and pelvic girdle for tenderness.

- Extensive palpation of the acute abdomen can be detrimental to the patient as well as delay transport; however, a hand placed gently on the abdomen can often detect rigidity suggestive of internal bleeding.

PERCUSSION

- Percussion can be a valuable inhospital evaluative tool, but has little or no field value.

Head-to-Toe Examination

Using the above assessment mechanisms, perform a rapid head-to-toe physical examination. The following is a systematic approach that can be used.

HEAD

- Check for lacerations, hematomas, bleeding, depressions.

FACE
- Check for cyanosis, pallor, flushing
- Look for blood from ears, nose, or mouth
- Look for broken teeth
- Note any obvious fracture of the jaw
- Check eye movement
- Look for diaphoresis

NECK
- Look at and palpate spine for tenderness, deformities, and rigidity
- Check neck veins for distension
- Check equality and quality of pulses
- Look for tracheal indrawing and deviation

CHEST
- Look for paradoxical chest movement
- Palpate thoracic cage for tenderness or deformity
- Check accessory muscles for indrawing
- Look for subcutaneous emphysema
- Note scars from previous chest or heart surgery
- Note barrel chest

BACK
- Note equality of chest movement
- Look for bruises, injuries, entry or exit wounds

ABDOMEN
- Look for bruises, penetrating injuries, distension
- Palpate gently for rigidity

PELVIS
- Palpate pelvic girdle for tenderness or deformity

EXTREMITIES
- Check pulses
- Palpate all extremities for tenderness or deformity
- Check for strength of hand grasp, sensations, and movement of all extremities
- Check color and capillary refill
- Look for deformities, needle marks

When performing a physical examination, place emphasis on areas pertinent to the chief complaint. Some medical conditions, such as myocardial infarction (MI), may not require so thorough a manipulative examination as that indicated for trauma. However, an abbreviated but systematic head-to-toe review of the body will organize your evaluation of the patient and at least ensure that no other problems exist.

In the abbreviated examination used for specific medical complaints, some aspects of the physical exam can be omitted. For example, you may not need to palpate the neck for deformity and tenderness in an MI patient, but you should look for distended neck veins.

Reporting to the Base Hospital

After patient assessment has been performed, a clear report of your findings must be transmitted to the base hospital. This is probably one of your most challenging duties, since communication is the basis for orders from the base hospital. If an order received is unusual or doesn't seem to fit the situation, review the information you have relayed to the hospital. In some areas, a code number is used to tactfully alert the physician that an order is in question. Misunderstandings between the hospital and the field are frequently the result of poor communication of assessment information.

Continually reassess your patient enroute, and inform the base hospital of any response to treatment or changes in patient status. Once you arrive at the hospital, be certain the physician or nurse who assumes care of your patient is informed *by you* of your observations and field treatments.

The concept of prehospital care is to stabilize life-threatening conditions and protect the patient from further injury until he can be seen in a medical facility. Therefore, it is imperative that prehospital assessment and stabilization be completed in the shortest possible time. Unnecessary field activities should be avoided, since they delay transport and thus can actually be detrimental to the patient.

ACUTE ABDOMINAL PAIN

There are two major categories of abdominal pain: traumatic and nontraumatic. Traumatic injuries can be *blunt,* e.g., being struck in the abdomen, or *penetrating,* e.g., a gunshot or knife wound. Blunt

11

trauma can be deceiving because there may not be bruises on the skin and internal damage can be far worse than external appearance suggests. Blunt abdominal trauma frequently causes internal hemorrhage, and a patient with no outward signs of trauma can quickly become cold, clammy, diaphoretic, pale, confused, and unconscious. Vital signs may be normal or they may confirm an internal disorder.

Penetrating abdominal trauma is similar to blunt trauma in that both can cause hemorrhagic shock. Both can also produce far greater internal damage than that shown on the body's surface. However, penetrating trauma can also cause external bleeding, which requires immediate control. Chest wounds below the nipple line must be suspected of having penetrated the abdomen.

In addition to traumatic injuries, a wide variety of medical conditions can create major abdominal pain, or abdominal pain of such sudden onset that emergency aid is requested. Included in these disorders are appendicitis, ulcers, herniation, pelvic inflammatory disease, dissecting abdominal aneurysm, ruptured ovarian cyst, ectopic pregnancy, and virtually countless others.

The clinical picture of abdominal pain is usually one of guarding, possibly with the knees drawn up toward the chest and the arms protecting the abdomen. The patient may be nauseated or may have vomited. He may have a history of either constipation or diarrhea, and might have obvious abdominal distension. Additionally, each of the possible clinical causes of the pain can have its own characteristic picture, such as the anxiety and knife-like tearing pain of the dissecting aneurysm.

Assessment of Abdominal Pain

Assessment should include attention to ABCs, a pertinent but brief medical history, a complete physical review for associated injuries, and a check of vital signs.

Don't evaluate the abdomen extensively. A hand placed gently on the abdomen may detect rigidity, suggesting internal bleeding. However, extensive palpation is of little value either to the patient, the paramedic, or the physician at the other end of the radio. Regardless of the findings, treatment will depend on other clinical signs such as those related to shock, and will not be altered by the results of a physical exam of the abdomen. More importantly, sophisticated palpation or auscultation of the abdomen will delay transportation, expose the patient to further trauma, and at the very least, cause unnecessary pain which will be repeated in the Emergency

Department (ED). There is always the possibility that an abdominal aneurysm is the cause of the pain, and it may not always present with an obvious pulsating mass. If an undetected abdominal aneurysm is palpated, it could rupture, subjecting the patient to possible exsanguination or death. The minimal data provided by extensive examination of the abdomen is not worth any of these consequences.

Field Treatment

Because of the great variety of possible causes of abdominal pain and the intensive diagnostic and laboratory tools that are required for an accurate identification of the source of the pain, the primary emphasis of field management is *not* differential diagnosis. The probability of immediate surgery is quite high, and very little actual treatment can be conducted in the field. Therefore, the paramedic should concentrate on assessing and stabilizing patient status, monitoring vital signs, and promptly transporting the patient to a medical facility for an appropriate work-up.

Field treatment of acute abdominal pain is essentially limited to 5% IV of 5% Dextrose in Water (D_5W) to keep open (TKO), or if shock is suspected, ringer's lactate (RL) or normal saline (NS) to replace fluid volume. If shock is profound, antishock trousers may be applied to restore vital signs. Penetrating objects should be stabilized and not removed unless Cardiopulmonary Resuscitation (CPR) is necessary or the antishock trousers are applied over the area of penetration.

Avoid giving medications, particularly narcotics or other analgesics. Don't give any food or fluids by mouth. Consider the patient's pain and take care during movement. Throughout the management of the run, move quickly and expeditiously to transport the patient without undue delay. Above all, be aware of the threat of shock, anticipate the signs, and recognize them when they appear. All patients in this category require oxygen, monitoring, and frequent assessment of vital signs. A nasogastric (NG) tube may be ordered to decompress the stomach. If the patient vomits or defecates, save a sample for the hospital.

AIRWAY OBSTRUCTION (FOREIGN BODY)

Patients with an upper airway obstruction will lose consciousness and experience cardiopulmonary arrest unless prompt intervention and correction of the obstruction is accomplished. Common causes of upper airway obstruction include the tongue, food, dentures, foreign bodies, emesis, blood clots, and broken teeth or bones. The obstruction may be either partial or complete. Patients with a partially obstructed airway should be left alone if they have good air exchange and a forceful cough. They can be given high-flow oxygen and transported promptly as long as they are able to breathe unassisted.

Good air exchange may progress quickly to poor exchange or total obstruction. Signs of increasing obstruction include an ineffective cough, inability to speak, inspiratory stridor or crowing, increasing respiratory difficulty and cyanosis, or unconsciousness. When a person with "cafe coronary" is unable to speak or cough and clutches the throat, he needs immediate intervention. Guidelines for the treatment of acute upper airway obstruction are as follows:

CONSCIOUS PATIENT

- *Effectively* attempting to clear his own airway, i.e., he can still talk and cough
    1. leave him alone
    2. offer reassurance
    3. encourage him to cough
    4. give high-flow oxygen if he will allow it
- *Ineffectively* attempting to clear his airway, i.e., he can no longer talk or cough
    1. administer four rapid back blows
    2. administer four rapid manual thrusts (chest or abdominal)
    3. repeat steps 1 and 2

UNCONSCIOUS PATIENT

1. open airway and attempt to ventilate
2. reposition head and attempt to ventilate again
3. try to remove the foreign body with Magill forceps and laryngoscope
4. if unsuccessful, or if Magill forceps are not immediately available, administer four back blows and four manual thrusts
5. repeat steps 2–4; if unsuccessful, transport as quickly as possible, using red lights and siren (Code 3) and continue series enroute

  6. consider cricothyrotomy if all other
   maneuvers fail

ANAPHYLACTIC SHOCK

 In a simple allergic reaction, the body reacts to a foreign substance, or antigen, by releasing histamine. This causes the characteristic rash, redness, swelling, and itching of allergy. Anaphylaxis is a severe allergic reaction, usually to an insect sting or a medication. In anaphylaxis, the release of histamine is more profound, causing the bronchial tree to constrict and go into spasm. Histamine also dilates the peripheral vessels and alters permeability of cell membranes, allowing escape of fluid volume into the tissue spaces.

 Acute anaphylaxis is usually an immediate response, but may be delayed from 10 to 30 minutes. The symptoms include sudden anxiety and restlessness, often with a pounding, or throbbing, headache. This is followed by a feeling of suffocation, a tightness in the chest, or actual cough or wheezing, due to bronchial constriction and can progress immediately to laryngeal edema and/or laryngospasm, profound peripheral vascular collapse, and respiratory failure. If treatment is not initiated promptly, death or permanent brain damage can result.

 The following steps can be taken in the field to treat anaphylactic shock. First, establish an airway, give oxygen and evaluate cardiorespiratory status. As rapidly as possible, administer 0.3 mg Epinephrine 1:1000 SC. Epinephrine is a drug with both alpha and beta properties; therefore, it acts to dilate the bronchial tree and constrict the vascular system when given in the recommended dose. Establish an IV of D₅W TKO in the event you may need to give other medications. Monitor vital signs and EKG frequently to determine the effectiveness of therapy.

 Following the administration of Epinephrine, Benadryl can be given to prevent further reaction by blocking histamine from the receptor sites. If the toxin was introduced through the skin, i.e., a bee sting or an injection, you may also administer 0.1 mg Epinephrine 1:1000 SC at the site of the reaction (if not a finger or toe) and/or use a constricting band proximal to the site if on an extremity. Both steps decrease the flow of toxin into the circulatory system. In an extremely severe reaction, additional drug therapy such as IV Epinephrine, dopamine, or Aminophylline may be required. Transport the patient with oxygen and pay close attention to vital signs.

BEHAVIORAL EMERGENCIES

A behavioral emergency exists when a patient demonstrates unusual, bizarre, or socially aberrant actions, ideas, or moods which may result in disruption to himself or those around him. These conditions can be caused by mental or emotional problems, but can also be a manifestation of an organic medical disorder. In the emergency setting it is important to rule out the presence of an acute medical condition before treating the patient as a behavioral disturbance.

Acute medical disorders which can mimic behavioral emergencies include head injuries, diabetic imbalance, hypoxia, or exposure to toxic substances. Depending on the particular patient situation, you may be able to eliminate some of these possibilities by giving oxygen or IV dextrose for differential diagnosis. However, in an emergency setting with an emotionally disturbed patient, it is often impractical to attempt such diagnostic maneuvers.

Behavioral emergencies caused by acute alterations in mental or emotional balance usually fall into one of four categories:

- *Acute Drug Intoxication:* Patients who have ingested depressants, amphetamines, hallucinogens, or other thought-altering agents.

- *Acute Alcohol Intoxication:* Patients who have ingested quantities of alcohol beyond the body's tolerance level.

- *Acute Psychiatric Disorders:* Patients exhibiting severe emotional distress, depressive states, manic states, schizophrenia, paranoia, hysterical conversion reaction, or catatonia.

- *Withdrawal Syndrome:* Patients in acute states of withdrawal from either alcohol or drugs.

Regardless of the cause of the behavioral disturbance, nearly all of these patients will fall into one of two behavioral categories when encountered in the field:

- *Quiet:* withdrawn, passive, or suicidal
- *Aggressive:* violent or combative.

The primary responsibility of the paramedic is to transport the patient for appropriate medical care rather than performing extensive psychiatric interview in the field. Therefore, field management of these patients consists of getting the patient into the ambulance and to the hospital expediently, while preventing either physical or emotional harm to the patient. Approach to treatment is determined by whether the patient is quiet or aggressive.

The Quiet Patient

The *quiet patient* may be suffering from acute grief, schizo-phrenia, ingestion of barbiturates or other depressive drugs, depres-sion, catatonia, hysterical conversion, manic states, or alcohol intoxication. Regardless of the cause, these patients respond best to a calm, direct manner, and active interest in their problem. An interested person who will provide support during this period of turmoil will often be able to stabilize the patient sufficiently to get him to the hospital. The suicidal patient usually is included in this group and requires special consideration because his situation is so acute that death may be imminent. Convey to the patient that you are intensely interested in his problem, and that you sincerely want to help him. Share your feelings and observations with him and try to convince him that you can help him deal with the situation. Avoid challenging commands, and don't underestimate or talk down to him. This type of patient is extremely perceptive; don't lie to him.

The Aggressive Patient

The *aggressive patient* presents more of a challenge to the paramedic than one who is quiet, because any action could result in further chaos as well as possible injury to others at the scene. Several principles can be employed in managing the violent patient. First, realize that the patient is protecting himself. Give him room. Don't make any moves that he may perceive as a threat. Use of body language is important with this type of patient. Don't stand between the patient and the door. Allow your body to assume a posture of relaxation, rather than confrontation. Don't stand directly in front of the patient; it is less threatening to sit or kneel off to one side. Allow the patient to vent his feelings. Use his own words to describe his situation. If all else fails, it may be necessary to forcefully restrain the patient. Once this decision is made, don't discuss it openly, just move in with at least four people and contain each extremity as rapidly as possible. Avoid yelling. Try to keep this action as calm as it can be. Keep the restraints on until you arrive at the hospital. Avoid a Code 3 response because this will further stimulate the patient.

General Guidelines

Behavioral emergencies require paramedics to use their instincts in order to manage the patient. Although several principles are available to assist you, it will be your own gut feelings that guide you in these situations. Sometimes a hand placed gently on the shoulder will give the patient the support and security he needs; other times, the same hand placed gently on the shoulder will be taken as a direct assault and will result in combative behavior. Keep in mind that your role is *not* to diagnose and solve the patient's problems; rather your primary goal is to get the patient safely and quickly to specialized medical care.

Several legal considerations are involved with behavioral emergencies. These include the validity of a consent form which is signed by an emotionally disturbed patient and the use of legal commitment to restrain and forcefully transport an unwilling patient. Learn the laws for your area and be aware of the resources available to you.

BURNS

The skin regulates fluid loss, controls temperature, prevents infection, and contains sensory receptors. Burns destroy some or all layers of skin, thus interfering with these important functions. The severity and treatment of a burn are determined by the degree, extent, and source of the burn.

The Degrees of Burns

A *first degree* burn is dry, painful, reddened, and blanches easily. It involves the epidermis only. A *second degree* burn has a moist surface, is red or mottled, has blisters, is painful, and blanches to pressure. It involves the epidermis and part of the dermis. *Third degree* burns are characterized as dry, hard and leathery, pearly white or charred, with congealed blood vessels and decreased pain secondary to destruction of nerve endings.

It is often quite difficult to determine the degree of the burn initially, but you should attempt to estimate it as accurately as possible. Regardless of the source of a burn, the degree is determined by the foregoing criteria.

The Extent of the Burn

The extent of a burn, i.e., the size of the area affected, is calculated in an adult by using the "Rule of Nines." This is a generalization of the percentage of body area involved. These percentage assignments, are illustrated in Figure 1.1.

The Sources of Burns

Three separate mechanisms can cause burns; they are heat, chemicals, and electrical current.

Thermal Burns

Any burn caused by heat, e.g., flame, steam, or liquid, is considered a thermal burn. When such burns occur skin layers, blood vessels, and nerve endings may be destroyed. In addition, the capillaries in the burned area are weakened and lose their permeability, allowing fluid and plasma proteins to escape from the circulatory system into the interstitial and extracellular spaces (the "third space"). If this displaced circulatory volume is not restored, hypovolemic shock will result.

Field management of thermal burns begins with the assurance that you and your patient are out of danger. Make sure the fire is extinguished and the clothing is not smoldering. Follow the ABCs with high-flow oxygen, determine whether or not there is respiratory involvement, and assess any associated injuries. Depending on the extent and degree of the burn, volume IV fluid replacement with RL, NS, or SPA may be indicated.

In minor first and second degree burns, saline soaks or ice packs may be beneficial in reducing pain. However, the ice should not be in direct contact with the skin, and the burn should never be soaked in ice water. Morphine Sulfate in small increments IV may be necessary for relief of pain if the patient doesn't respond to reassurance and other basic measures.

Keep the patient warm to avoid hypothermia; wrap in clean sheets and transport. Frequent evaluation of vital signs and respiratory status is important, as is a good history and physical examination. Remove all rings, watches, necklaces, and other constrictive articles. Don't give any fluids orally. Don't apply any grease or ointment to the burns, don't break any blisters, and don't remove any clothing that is stuck to burned tissue. Do not administer any medications by the IM route.

Chemical Burns

Chemical burns cause a pathological state similar to thermal burns, but are usually more localized. Basically, these burns are

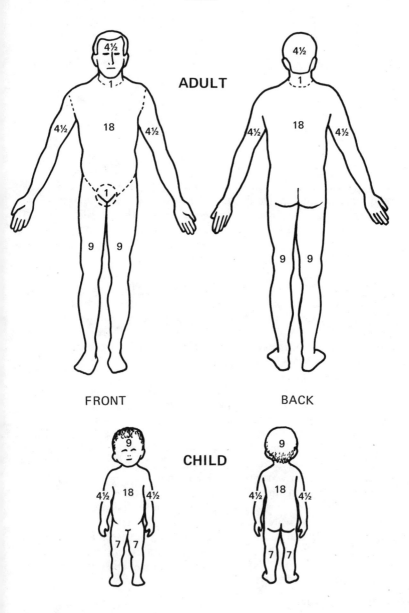

Figure 1.1 Refer to the Rule of Nines when estimating body surface area involvement of burn injuries.

treated the same as a thermal injury, except that the chemical must first be removed by flushing with copious amounts of water. Because the chemical can continue burning for some time, the area must be flushed continuously during transport. If large body areas are involved, the patient should be placed in a shower or hosed off. If the chemical is a dry powder, brush off as much as possible before hosing the patient with water. Remove clothing carefully to prevent further exposure to the chemical.

Electrical Burns

Electrical burns are unique because there is a danger of internal damage along the pathways of the electrical current. Respiratory arrest or ventricular fibrillation can occur secondary to the electrical current itself. Field treatment follows the same principles as that of thermal burns, but with emphasis on respiratory and cardiovascular support. Always start an IV and monitor EKG as a precautionary measure. Electrical burns are very serious and should always be transported to the hospital for evaluation.

Complications of Burn Injuries

Respiratory Involvement

Many burn patients have associated respiratory involvement which further complicates their injury. Early recognition of pulmonary burns is essential. Pulmonary involvement should be suspected if the burn occurs within an enclosed area, involves the face or neck, or results in singed facial and nasal hairs or soot or blisters in the nose, mouth, or oropharynx. Initially, a patient with respiratory involvement may have normal respirations, but as burn edema and bronchial irritation increase, signs and symptoms of dyspnea, hoarseness, cough, and cyanosis may be seen. Do not use MS if pulmonary involvement is suspected, and be prepared to intubate if laryngeal edema is anticipated. Give high-flow oxygen and transport promptly.

Carbon Monoxide Poisoning

Carbon monoxide (CO) poisoning should be suspected in all patients found unconscious at the scene of a fire, or any patient burned in an enclosed area. Signs and symptoms include headache, weakness, tingling in the extremities, confusion, reckless behavior, collapse, and coma. Cyanosis can be masked because of the effect carbon monoxide has on the mucous membranes. The cherry-red coloring often attributed to CO poisoning is a late characteristic, and thus is an unreliable field sign. Treatment for CO poisoning is to remove the patient from the source of the gas and then hyperventilate with high-flow oxygen to help blow off the carbon monoxide.

Other Complications

While *infection* is a leading cause of death following a major burn, it generally does not appear for 24–48 hours. In the field, you can help prevent this complication by keeping the burned area as clean as possible. Another complication is *corneal abrasion,* which frequently occurs following flash burns of the face. Signs and symptoms include a scratchy feeling, blurred vision, or clouding of the cornea. Treatment consists of saline irrigation, closing the eyes and keeping them still, and application of dry dressings.

Transporting Burn Patients

You will frequently be in a position to witness patients with very minor burns which do not need to be rushed to a hospital, but instead can be seen by a private physician. However, some burns can appear minor but still need immediate specialized care to prevent longterm disability or even death. As a general rule, patients requiring transport are those with:

- Second and third degree burns over 15–30% of the body
- Involvement of critical areas (hands, face, feet, genitalia)
- Respiratory involvement
- Associated soft tissue injury and/or fractures
- Electrical injuries
- Very young or very old patients

CARDIOGENIC SHOCK

Like all forms of shock, cardiogenic shock is basically a condition in which perfusion levels are inadequate for body functions. This form of shock results from the heart's inability to pump efficiently. It is most often caused by a massive MI, but can also be caused by sustained tachyarrhythmias, pericardial tamponade, end-stage congestive heart failure (CHF) with pulmonary edema, massive pulmonary embolus, tension pneumothorax, or valvular disease. As the heart loses its ability to contract effectively, the cardiac output drops and triggers the release of catecholamines. This results in cool, clammy skin, diaphoresis, and tachycardia. Despite these compensatory mechanisms, cerebral oxygenation remains inadequate and mental sluggishness and confusion are apparent. The most characteristic feature of this type of shock is the early appearance of hypotension.

Field Management of Cardiogenic Shock

Inhospital management is directed at treating the specific cause of the disorder. If the cause is readily apparent in the field, it should be managed prior to treating the shock state. In the field, cardiogenic shock is most often seen in association with MI or CHF, and requires treatment directed toward maintaining vital body functions. Since this form of shock is not caused by fluid loss, the patient does not need IV fluid replacement in the field. To give excessive fluids would cause an undue workload on an already taxed heart, and would contribute to patient deterioration.

The treatment of choice is dopamine to increase the heart's effectiveness and raise the blood pressure. If dopamine is unavailable, vasopressors should be given. Also, high-flow oxygen and other supportive measures must be instituted. The patient may have suffered myocardial damage and therefore needs to be closely monitored with antiarrhythmic therapy as needed.

Unfortunately, cardiogenic shock carries an 80%-90% mortality rate despite aggressive medical attention. However, many clinicians feel that early administration of dopamine is beginning to reduce this figure. This type of patient warrants critical attention and prompt transport.

CEREBROVASCULAR ACCIDENT

Cerebrovascular accident (CVA), also referred to as stroke, is a result of a thrombus, embolus, or hemorrhage which occludes the blood supply to a portion of the brain causing ischemia and/or infarction. Subsequent signs and symptoms are related to the area of the brain where the damage has occurred. Contributing factors include hypertension, atherosclerosis, thrombi, emboli, aneurysms, intracranial masses, and the use of birth control pills or anticoagulants. The patient's history may also include chronic atrial fibrillation or myocardial infarction.

Assessment includes a thorough history and physical examination which will frequently direct the treatment. CVAs are usually of sudden onset and may have been preceded by a headache. In the immediate postinjury stage, the blood pressure usually remains high, but may possibly be in the normal, or low range. Other signs and symptoms include unilateral paralysis and/or muscle weakness, aphasia, drooping of the mouth, drooling, incontinence, and occasionally unconsciousness or unequal pupils. The patient may have central respiratory involvement but this phenomenon is rare. Assessment should include an examination for associated injuries.

A disorder similar to CVA is transient ischemic attack (TIA). This condition is caused by cerebral vascular spasms or microemboli which produce many of the same symptoms as a CVA. TIA differs from CVA only in that its effects are temporary. The patient with TIA may be fully recovered by the time medical help arrives. Even though the patient may appear asymptomatic, all suspected TIAs should be transported for further medical evaluation, as it may be indicative of impending CVA.

Management of TIA and CVA

There is no relevant difference in management of symptomatic TIA and CVA patients in the prehospital setting. Airway control may require the insertion of an oral or nasopharyngeal airway and suction should be readily available. Postitioning the patient on his side will further reduce the chances of aspiration. Oxygen should be administered to combat any associated hypoxia. An IV will probably be ordered at a slow rate to keep the vein open in case medications are needed. Frequent reassessment of vital signs, neurological status, and level of consciousness are necessary during transport.

CHEST TRAUMA

Accidents frequently result in trauma to the chest; therefore, they may affect the respiratory and/or cardiovascular systems.

Traumatic Pneumothorax/Hemothorax

Traumatic pneumothorax/hemothorax occurs when either air or blood enter the pleural cavity following trauma, resulting in a partial or complete collapse of one or both lungs. These disorders are common complications of chest trauma, particularly fractured ribs, and usually render the patient dyspneic. Other signs include bruising of the chest wall and crepitus in the affected area. Often associated with the severe dyspnea is pain on inspiration and guarded respirations. Upon auscultation, breath sounds may be diminished on the affected side or increased on the opposite side depending on the extent of lung involvement. Subcutaneous emphysema may also be present. Field treatment is directed toward supporting respirations and preventing shock. Give high-flow oxygen, apply the monitor, check the patient for associated injuries and immobilize as needed. Start an IV of RL or NS for possible volume replacement. Assist ventilations as necessary and watch patient closely for possible progression to tension pneumothorax.

Tension Pneumothorax

Tension pneumothorax is created by an opening in the chest with a one-way flap that allows air to enter the pleural cavity with each breath, but does not allow air to be expired. This alters intrathoracic pressure and creates an internal tension which increases with each breath. This condition should be suspected when a patient becomes increasingly dyspneic and anxious with each respiration. As the condition progresses, more air fills the affected side, and the trachea may shift to the opposite side along with the mediastinum. If allowed to continue, the pressure can compress the good lung and hinder respirations. This tension causes the heart and great vessels to be shifted and compressed, thus altering circulatory status by preventing blood from returning to the heart.

Although tension pneumothorax can be fatal if left untreated, it rarely progresses to a life-threatening stage in less time than it takes to transport the patient. Therefore, it may be more appropriate to transport the patient than to initiate invasive field treatment unless the transport time is unusually long. If the patient is suffering from tension pneumothorax and requires immediate relief, a needle thoracostomy may be ordered. This involves inserting a cannula with an attached flutter valve through the affected chest wall and into the pleural space to allow internal and external pressures to equalize. Assist respirations as needed, monitor vital signs and EKG, and transport promptly.

Flail Chest

Occasionally, trauma to the chest will fracture several contiguous ribs, thus creating a floating section which prevents the chest wall from adequately expanding for ventilation. The patient will exhibit extreme anxiety with dyspnea, tachycardia, and possible cyanosis. Paradoxical respirations will be present resulting in impaired respiratory function. Treatment is aimed at stabilizing the chest wall with support to the injured side in order to facilitate ventilation. This can best be done by placing the victim on the injured side and/or splinting the affected side with sandbags. Following this, the patient should be ventilated with a positive-pressure resuscitator and intubated if necessary. Check the patient for associated injuries, immobilize the spine, monitor cardiac and respiratory status, and start an IV of RL or NS. Volume replacement may be necessary if hypovolemia is present. Watch the patient closely for evidence of progression to tension pneumothorax and transport immediately.

Open Chest Injuries

If there is a penetrating injury to the chest wall, air is likely to enter the pleural cavity and cause extreme respiratory distress, cyanosis, and a sucking sound with each inspiration. A common treatment for this "sucking chest wound" is to seal it with a Vasoline gauze dressing. However, this might convert the injury into a tension pneumothorax. If the patient becomes increasingly dyspneic following application of the dressing, remove the dressing to allow release of internal pressure; then reseal the wound. Support respiratory and cardiovascular status as necessary and transport quickly. If a penetrating object is protruding from the wound, leave it in place and stabilize it with bandages. However, should CPR or antishock trousers become necessary, the protruding object will have to be removed to prevent further damage.

Cardiac Trauma

Cardiac trauma very often accompanies chest trauma. Frequently, the only early warning of cardiac trauma is a suspicious mechanism of injury, i.e., chest impact with a steering wheel or dashboard. Other signs which may substantiate your findings include rib fractures or bruising over the pericardium. Some of the more common types of cardiac trauma are discussed in the following paragraphs.

Cardiac Contusion

Cardiac contusion occurs from direct blunt trauma to the heart, and can present as cardiac insufficiency or a myocardial infarction.

The patient may complain of chest pain, and the EKG can reveal ST changes or arrhythmias. Treatment includes high-flow oxygen and support of vital functions. Due to possible ventricular damage, arrhythmias are likely and should be treated as necessary with antiarrhythmic agents. Consider the possibility of an underlying MI in addition to any presenting trauma.

Ventricular Rupture

Ventricular rupture, or trauma to the great vessels, can cause rapid exsanguination and profound circulatory collapse. This situation requires massive volume restoration with IV volume expanders and antishock trousers. Resuscitation of a patient with injuries of this nature is very unlikely.

Pericardial Tamponade

Pericardial tamponade occurs when blood accumulates in the pericardial space and suppresses the pumping action of the heart. This condition usually results from either blunt or penetrating trauma to the chest wall. Signs and symptoms include tachycardia, hypotension, distension of neck veins, cyanosis, muffled heart sounds, and profound shock. Immediate pericardiocentesis is the treatment of choice. If you are medically or legally unauthorized to perform this procedure in the field, transport immediately and support vital functions enroute.

CONGESTIVE HEART FAILURE

Congestive heart failure (CHF) occurs when the heart loses its ability to eject blood effectively, thus resulting in pulmonary and/or peripheral engorgement. Many patients who suffer MI, valvular disease, or hypertension are apt to experience varying degrees of mechanical heart failure at some stage of their disease. Often it is the left ventricle that fails initially, while the right continues to eject blood normally. As blood volume increases on the left side, pressure increases and there is a backup of fluids into the pulmonary vasculature and the alveoli. This accumulation of fluid in the alveoli is called pulmonary edema. Signs and symptoms of left heart failure and its associated pulmonary edema include restlessness, tachycardia, dyspnea, fatigue, orthopnea, paroxysmal nocturnal dyspnea, cyanosis, diaphoresis, rales, and in severe cases, pink frothy sputum. The restlessness, anxiety, and feeling of suffocation associated with left heart failure are due to hypoxia.

Field Treatment of CHF

Field treatment is aimed at relief of pulmonary engorgement and reoxygenation. Reassure these patients and allow them to remain in a sitting position. Administer high-flow oxygen; use prongs if the mask is resisted. When severe pulmonary edema is present, positive pressure ventilation should be attempted in an effort to drive fluid out of the alveoli. Start an IV D_5W TKO as a line for drug administration. Drug therapy includes morphine sulphate to help alleviate anxiety and pool venous blood by peripheral vasodilatation. Digoxin can be used to increase contractility of the heart and slow the rate. Lasix is given to reduce circulating volume, thereby decreasing venous return to the heart. Aminophylline can be used to decrease respiratory effort by dilating the bronchioles. It also decreases venous return because it acts as a vasodilator and a mild diuretic.

If the patient is in severe distress, rotating tourniquets may be applied prior to or in conjunction with drug therapy. They act to decrease venous return to the heart, thereby decreasing myocardial workload. When tourniquets are used, evaluate arterial pulses after each application and rotate systematically. Monitor the patient, watching closely for tachyarrhythmias and hypoxia-induced ectopic beats.

Right ventricular failure commonly follows left ventricular failure due to pulmonary hypertension. Classic signs and symptoms of right-sided heart failure include distended neck veins, peripheral edema, liver engorgement, and ascites. Other than its association with left ventricular failure, isolated right failure has minimal implication for the paramedic because it is not treated in the field.

DIABETES

Diabetes is a relative imbalance between body sugar and insulin levels, resulting in cellular deprivation of glucose. All body cells need sugar to perform metabolism; without it, tissues will die. A few central organs, especially the brain, have a more acute need for sugar and will die very quickly if deprived of it. Sugar is usually obtained from foods, and is distributed to the tissues in the blood stream. Insulin, a hormone normally produced in the pancreas, enables the glucose to leave the bloodstream and cross over the cell wall to be used by the cell. This process can be upset in one of two ways: 1) lack of sugar causes the blood sugar level to drop, resulting in hypoglycemia; or 2) lack of insulin prevents the glucose from crossing over the cell wall, so it remains in the blood stream and results in hyperglycemia.

These are the two extremes of imbalance in diabetes, but a patient can experience any stage between. The symptoms are complex, can overlap one another, and are very often indistinguishable. It is frequently difficult to accurately differentiate between hyperglycemia and hypoglycemia in the field, particularly if the patient is unconscious. Regardless of which imbalance is present, a generalized field treatment can be given if the specific state can't be identified.

Hypoglycemia

The most critical of the two diabetic extremes is hypoglycemia, since sugar is needed immediately to keep the brain alive. This condition may occur if patients eat less than their usual diet, increase their activities abruptly, suffer from injury or a febrile illness, or accidentally take too much insulin. Such patients appear to have fainted, or feel very weak, and exhibit cool, moist skin. Vital signs are relatively normal. If the patients are alert, they will be extremely nervous, or they may be unconscious or even experience seizures. Hypoglycemia often causes transient personality changes: Patients may appear hostile, aggressive, or exhibit bizarre behavior. This can cause patients to be mistakenly labeled drunk when they are really hypoglycemic.

Hyperglycemia

In contrast, hyperglycemia has a slower onset of symptoms and the patient appears very ill. This condition can be caused by inadequate production of natural insulin, by skipping an insulin dose, or by eating an unusually large amount of food. Patients might have hot, flushed skin, fruity-smelling breath, rapid weak pulse, low blood pressure, signs of dehydration, and may present with deep Kussmaul respirations. If patients are still alert, they may complain of extreme thirst.

Treating the Diabetic

To aid in diagnosing an unconscious patient as a diabetic, you should search for Medic–alert tags or cards on or about the patient. Check for oral hypoglycemic agents, insulin preparations, syringes, or urine-testing materials. Examine the patient for injection sites, usually on the anterior thigh or abdomen. If the patient is older or has had the disease for some time, the legs may show signs of poor circulation including amputations of digits or legs, and the eyes may be clouded by cataracts.

If the clinical signs don't distinctly identify the problem, or if the condition is determined to be hypoglycemia, the patient must be given sugar in the most appropriate form. You needn't worry about giving sugar to undiagnosed patients because it won't hurt those who need insulin, and it may be vital to the survival of those who need sugar.

In the diabetic patient who is still conscious and has a gag reflex, administer 7 oz Glucola orally. If he is unconscious or losing consciousness, start an IV of RL, NS, or D₅W TKO, and follow it with a bolus of D₅₀W IV push. Severe dehydration frequently accompanies hyperglycemia, so you may be ordered to begin volume replacement. For those patients in whom an IV is not possible, you should administer one-half tube of Instant Glucose Paste orally between the cheek and gums; position the patient to avoid aspiration. Always try to draw a blood sample for a baseline blood sugar level before giving any form of glucose.

As with other chronically ill patients, diabetics occasionally call for treatment and then refuse transportation after being stabilized. Stress to these patients the importance of being reevaluated medically since they may require changes in their management. If they still refuse transportation, refer them to their private physician and be sure to get a release form signed.

DROWNING

The pathophysiology of near-drowning is altered by the type of water in which the patient was immersed, and clinical conditions will vary depending on whether the water was salt, fresh, clean, dirty, or chlorinated. However, none of these factors will affect prehospital management. Therefore, discussion of this syndrome can be simplified.

The major clinical problems found in the near-drowning patient are hypoxia and acidosis. These are attributed to the common occurrence of aspiration of water and/or vomitus into the lungs, and the subsequent compromised respiratory exchange. Generally, the status of a near-drowning patient will be affected by the length of time submerged, age, concurrent injuries, and previous medical condition.

Field Management of Asymptomatic Near-Drowning Patients

Following recovery from the water, the asymptomatic patient may appear stable and deny any distress. However, the onset of hypoxia, cyanosis, pulmonary edema, and lung complications may appear minutes or hours later. For this reason it is essential that all near-drowning patients be watched closely and examined at a medical facility. Field treatment includes high-flow oxygen, a thorough exam for associated injuries, an IV of D_5W TKO, and monitoring of EKG.

Field Management of Symptomatic Near-Drowning Patients

The symptomatic patient is most often in cardiac arrest and should be treated in much the same way as any other arrest situation. This would include CPR and prompt airway management with an esophageal or endotracheal airway. Ventilation should be with high-concentration oxygen under pressure. An IV of D_5W TKO is necessary to ensure a line for medications such as sodium bicarbonate and antiarrhythmics. Dopamine or vasopressors may be necessary to support cardiovascular status.

When resuscitating a near-drowning victim, do not waste time trying to clear the lungs of water. Anticipate that the patient may vomit, and proceed to pass a nasogastric tube or position the patient to prevent additional aspiration.

Assess the patient for associated injuries. It is not uncommon for the near-drowning victim to have concurrent spinal cord or head injuries, so immediate stabilization is required even before removing the victim from the water. Consider the possibility that a medical condition might have caused the accident. Attempt to rule out MI, anaphylaxis from jellyfish or stingray injury, or pulmonary injury following a diving accident.

Keep the patient warm and monitor closely for EKG or vital sign changes. Collect a specimen of the water and take it with you to the hospital for analysis. Continue respiratory and cardiovascular support.

ENVIRONMENTAL EMERGENCIES

Snakebite

It has been estimated that in nearly 25% of all bites from poisonous snakes *no* venom has been released, so you must first determine whether or not the snake actually has injected venom with its bite. Indications that this has occurred include rapid onset (within 3–10 minutes) of pain, redness, and swelling at the site. The severity of response to envenomation is determined by the intensity of symptoms and how quickly they appear following the bite. These can be influenced by the size and type of the snake, the size of the patient, how much venom the snake injected, whether or not the bite penetrated the vascular system, and the general medical condition of the patient. Children will always be more severely affected because of the proportionately large amount of venom injected.

Pit Vipers

The venom of pit vipers (including rattlesnakes, water moccasins, and copperheads) destroys red blood cells, interferes with coagulation, and destroys body tissues. When reporting to the base hospital, it is important to differentiate between local and systemic symptoms, since these categories will be used to grade the severity of the reaction. Local symptoms include pain, redness, and swelling at the site. General systemic symptoms include sustained tachycardia and tachypnea, tingling around the mouth, shortness of breath, weakness, faintness, nausea, and muscle tremors. These can progress quickly to hematemesis, hematuria, respiratory depression, and coma. In extreme cases, death can occur within an hour.

As soon as you suspect envenomation, calm the patient, sit him down, and do not allow him to move; any movement at all will further circulate the venom. Place a constricting band just proximal to the site, adjusting it to occlude venous return, but ensuring that an arterial pulse is palpable in the extremity. Keep the affected limb below the level of the heart to delay absorption. If you arrive within 10 minutes after envenomation and the hospital is more than an hour away, you may be ordered to make two small incisions over the fang marks. These should be parallel to the extremity if possible, and about ⅛ to ¼ inch deep (down to the venom), and no more than about ¼ inch long. Apply suction and continue during transport.

You will probably be ordered to start an IV of D_5W TKO, and to watch respiratory and cardiovascular status closely. Monitor EKG and report any changes in patient status. Analgesics are contraindicated for snakebites because they can aggravate some of the symptoms. Ice has long been used to slow down circulation in the area and to help reduce pain. However, ice itself can cause tissue necrosis, and should only be used if wrapped in cloth to protect the tissues. Never soak the limb in ice water, as extensive damage can result. When you transport these patients, they must be carried to the ambulance; do not allow them to walk.

Coral Snakes

Another category of poisonous snakes is the coral snake group, whose highly toxic venom can cause death by paralysis if not treated immediately. As with pit vipers, the symptoms can range from mild to severe, and may be local or systemic. Systemic symptoms are primarily neurologic, and may not appear for as long as 18 hours after the bite.

Once it is established that envenomation has actually occurred, begin treatment promptly. Field treatment is the same as the treatment of pit viper injuries.

Marine Animals

Marine animals, such as stingray and jellyfish, cause minor wounds with major pain. The pain of a stingray injury can frequently be reduced by using hot packs or soaking in hot water. The venom of these animals is heat-labile, so the application of heat detoxifies the protein substance. The sites of jellyfish stings should be washed with alcohol. This deactivates the microorganisms on the skin and prevents them from further discharge. Pour the alcohol over the affected skin and leave it on 6–8 minutes. If available, apply a baking soda paste and allow it to dry. Remember that both of these animals can cause allergic response, and anaphylaxis is a possibility. Watch for signs of systemic response to the injury.

Spider Bites

The two spiders which most commonly cause problems are the Black Widow and the Brown Recluse, or Violin Spider. Bites of these spiders are usually identified by small, painful red blebs associated with general symptoms ranging from gastrointestinal upset to anaphylaxsis. A good history and physical exam will facilitate proper diagnosis. Specific antidotes are available for common poisonous bites, so prompt transport is indicated. During transport, monitor the patient closely and support vital body functions as required.

Heat Injuries

Heat exposure occurs when a person is exposed to hot climates for an extended length of time. It can result in many symptoms commonly found with sunburn. Along with the burned and blistered areas of the skin, generalized manifestations such as fever, chills, and malaise are common.

Heat Cramps

Heat cramps can be found with or without other symptoms of heat exposure. These are muscle cramps caused by salt loss following profuse sweating. The patient has a normal temperature and needs salt to rebalance body fluids. If the heat exposure is allowed to persist untreated, the patient will deteriorate to heat exhaustion and/or heat stroke. Treatment of minor heat exposure is supportive, but includes cooling measures, change of environment, and possible oral administration of salt enriched fluids.

Heat Exhaustion

Extremes of heat exposure will result in heat exhaustion. The patient displays normal temperature, but with accompanying signs such as cramps, nausea, vomiting, thirst, and in extreme cases, shock. Dehydration should be corrected with an IV of RL or NS, and the patient should be cooled gently.

Heat Stroke

If allowed to continue, heat exhaustion will progress to heat stroke. This is a true medical emergency resulting from heat damage to the brain's temperature regulatory center. At this point, perspiration ceases and the body temperature rises causing hot, dry, flushed skin. The pulse is full, and the blood pressure may be low, normal or high. Systemic signs include vertigo, headache, convulsions, ataxia, vomiting, diarrhea, abdominal pain, and coma. Treatment must include rapid cooling measures and change of environment. In addition, an IV of RL or NS, oxygen, control of seizures, and supportive measures should be instituted as necessary. This patient should be closely monitored. Death can occur from either irreversible failure of the temperature regulator in the hypothalamus, or by heart failure from the increased workload.

Cold Injuries

The occurrence and severity of cold injuries will depend on the length of exposure, actual temperature reading, humidity, conductive environmental factors, and wind velocities. *General body* cooling progresses from shivering, listlessness, and apathy to unconsciousness and death. Management includes change of environment, observation of vital signs, controlled heat application, and dry clothing.

Local cold damage, or frostbite, is classified by degrees, as are burns. Field treatment consists of gentle warming, dry wraps, and dressing of blistered areas. Do not allow affected part to cool again; don't start rewarming if you won't be able to keep the part warm. Evaluate the circulatory status of the affected part at frequent intervals.

Radiation

Radiation signs depend on the amount of body exposed, length of exposure, strength and type of radiation, distance from the source, and amount of shielding. Susceptibility to injury is greater in rapidly dividing cells as in young infants, and in undifferentiated cells found in sex organs. Symptoms include malaise, fever, nausea, vomiting, and diarrhea. Treat symptomatically and avoid personal exposure.

MAJOR TRAUMA AND TRIAGE

Major trauma situations are perhaps the most challenging emergency the paramedic will encounter. Included in this category are single patients with major or multiple injuries, and groups of patients, some of whom might have multiple injuries. The scene is often chaotic since many things have to be done at one time, and often there will be more than one top priority. Organization of activities is often difficult and yet it is essential to effective utilization of personnel and optimum management of life-threatening injuries.

Major Trauma to a Single Patient

Trauma often involves vital body organs, or more than one body system. When it does, it is considered life-threatening and requires immediate attention. Included in this category are major head, chest, or abdominal wounds, multisystem trauma, and fractures of large vascular bones such as the femur and pelvis.

When faced with major trauma, the complexity of the patient's problems may cause you to move without thinking. To avoid this, keep the basic ABCs in mind and follow them in patient management. If you can control ABCs, you won't need to worry about the other manifestations until you get the patient to the hospital.

35

AIRWAY	• Look for structural defects, such as fractured mandible external trauma to the trachea, open chest wounds, or flail chest. (If present, correct with positioning, bandaging, or splinting.
	• Consider the possibility of spinal cord injury and immobilize spine if possible.)

Check for obstruction which can be caused by blood, bone fragments, tooth chips, or swelling; use suctioning, positioning, and airways as needed

BREATHING	• Ascertain that the patient is breathing; if not, ventilate
	• Administer supplemental oxygen; assist ventilations as needed
	• Look for breathing patterns that might include periods of apnea and can indicate inadequate exchange
BLEEDING	• Rapidly survey the body and control major external bleeding
CIRCULATION	• If circulation is absent, initiate CPR and standard resuscitative measures
	• Support blood pressure with IV fluid volume replacement
	• Assess perfusion; consider antishock trousers
	• Monitor EKG; treat arrhythmias as appropriate
	• It is unlikely that drugs would be required in a multiple trauma patient

After managing initial priorities, prepare to transport. Immobilize the patient, bandage and splint injuries as required, and reassess vital signs frequently. Do not give analgesics or oral fluids. This patient will probably require the specialized care available at a regional trauma center.

Multiple-Patient Situations

The problems of the single patient with multiple injuries can be so complex as to intimidate even the most experienced paramedic. When there are more than one of these trauma patients, all of the problems are compounded. In the multi-casualty situation you must consider the number of patients, available manpower, the extent and severity of injuries, and the ages and medical conditions of the patients in order to determine the complexity of the situation and set priorities to manage it.

After assessing the scene and the capabilities of your team, you must exercise leadership and respond with appropriate degree of urgency, judgment, and skill to deal with the problems at hand. Call for backup as soon as the need is identified. Make sure the directions you give to other rescue personnel are clear and concise; leave no room for misunderstandings.

In a multiple-patient incident, it is essential that a single individual be identified as *triage officer* to direct patient management without confusion and duplication. The radio man is usually in the best position to accept this responsibility. In this role, the radio man will direct the patient man and other personnel, communicate with the hospital, and coordinate all patient management.

A nonmedical person, usually the highest ranking fire department official, can be assigned to control the nonmedical aspects of the scene. This person will be responsible for coordination of ambulances and other emergency vehicles, fire suppression, crowd control, and rescue activities.

On arrival at a multi-casualty incident, set up a communications base in a safe place near access to ambulances. If the patients are scattered, have them gathered to this central location near the radio man. The radio man must immediately perform a 30-second survey of each patient, then assign each patient an identification (ID) number and a priority for care and/or transportation. In triaging, you must attempt to do the most good for the most people. Categories for priority of care are:

1. IMMEDIATE   airway, respiratory problems, major bleeding problems

2. URGENT   head, chest, or abdominal injuries, major or multiple fractures, multisystem injuries (this category has limited field treatment and requires immediate transport)

3. MINIMAL   minor injuries

4. DELAYED full arrest situations following trauma (resuscitation rate is very low; care of salvagable patients must take priority; do not initiate CPR or treatment unless adequate manpower is available)

In order to minimize confusion, only the radio man should communicate with the base hospital. Compile a separate record for each patient and use it to organize radio reports. Report on the most serious patients first, using the ID numbers for clarity. Have the base hospital inventory the availability of resources at area hospitals and direct patients to hospitals which have the capabilities for handling their specific injuries.

The radio man accompanied by the patient man, should conduct the initial review of each patient and identify the most life-threatening injuries; the patient man is then directed to institute appropriate measures with that patient. In multiple trauma situations, this is generally confined to ABCs, and rarely gets more sophisticated than an IV and/or antishock trousers. The patient man should utilize available personnel as much as possible to assist with patient management. Since most care in these situations is basic life support, the paramedic is best utilized to delegate, coordinate, and oversee the care given by others.

In preparing to transport, a paramedic should fill each ambulance according to the capabilities of the hospital it is going to. For example, if ambulance A is going to a hospital which has a trauma center and a burn unit, those patients with major trauma and/or burns should be placed in ambulance A, rather than ambulance B, which is going to a small community hospital with limited resources and no surgical staff available. Ambulance B should be filled with patients in the ambulatory category, who will be most likely to receive adequate care at the smaller hospital.

Be certain that all treatment records are securely affixed to the patient. In casualty situations with many victims, it may be necessary to transport a patient with an IV in an ambulance without advanced life support (ALS) personnel to monitor the solution. This is not an acceptable standard in conventional circumstances, and should be avoided if at all possible, but it may be necessary if the number of critical patients exceeds the available manpower resources.

MYOCARDIAL INFARCTION (MI)

Myocardial infarction (MI) is defined as the death of a portion of the heart muscle, most often due to occlusion of a coronary artery by plaque buildup or a thrombus. The usual presentation includes severe substernal chest pain which is a clinical manifestation of myocardial anoxia. The patient may deny actual pain, but will refer to it instead as pressure, indigestion, or a crushing sensation that came on suddenly which may have radiated down one or both arms or up into the neck or jaw. Other signs and symptoms include cold, clammy skin, diaphoresis, and nausea or vomiting. Depending on the severity of the damage, the patient may also have evidence of CHF and/or cardiogenic shock due to decreased effectiveness of the left ventricle.

The patient with an MI is subject to a wide range of arrhythmias which may be the result of either direct injury to the conduction system or underlying myocardial hypoxia. These arrhythmias can range from sinus bradycardia to ventricular fibrillation, and are the leading cause of death in this type of patient. Because the MI patient has such potential for lethal arrhythmias it is imperative that you connect him to a cardiac monitor immediately, and promptly treat any arrhthymias that have the potential to cause a drop in cardiac output. Premature ventricular contractions and ventricular tacycardia are commonly seen in association with MIs and should be treated with lidocaine immediately. You should also consider the prophylactic use of lidocaine in the field management of all MI patients to prevent primary ventricular fibrillation. Watch for bradycardias and heart blocks as the sinoatrial (SA) and atrio-ventricular (AV) nodes may be temporarily damaged. If atropine is required, it should be used cautiously since an excessive increase in heart rate can cause extension of the infarction.

Treatment of MI

Any patient with chest pain should be treated as a myocardial infarction until proven otherwise. Administer oxygen at a high-flow rate to increase oxygen supply to the heart, but be cautious with patients with chronic lung disease. Start an IV TKO as a lifeline for possible medications. Morphine sulfate can be given in small increments to help relieve the pain and reduce the patient's anxiety. It is important to calm the patient as soon as possible to prevent any undue workload on the heart. Take vital signs as needed with particular emphasis on heart rate and blood pressure. If you detect hypotension, the patient has probably developed cardiogenic shock and may require dopamine or vasopressors. Frequent assessment of lung sounds is also essential because the patient with a large MI can progress very rapidly to CHF and pulmonary edema.

When preparing for transport, don't allow the patient to walk to the guerney. Keep the oxygen on enroute, and avoid a Code 3 response. Continue to reassure the patient, because this disorder is often accompanied by a feeling of impending death.

NEUROLOGICAL EMERGENCIES

Assessment

Neurological emergencies generally present as interruptions in the normal motor or sensory capabilities of the brain, spinal column, or peripheral nerves. The threat to life associated with head injuries and other neurological disorders is a result of the rapid or insidious buildup of pressure within the skull as blood or fluid accumulates. This increase in intracranial pressure can result in displacement of the brain stem, causing rapid deterioration of the patient's condition. Signs and symptoms of increased intracranial pressure include decreased level of consciousness, changes in vital signs, respiratory depression, and nonreactive pupil(s).

It is important to perform an accurate and rapid neurological assessment initially so that any changes can be identified during subsequent evaluations. The neurological assessment should include an evaluation of the following:

1. Are there any abnormal respiratory patterns?
2. What is the level of consciousness?
   - Can the patient open eyes on command?
   - If so, is he oriented to time, place, and person?
   - Does the patient respond to touch or to deep pain?
   - If so, is the response appropriate, inappropriate, or neurologically abnormal?
3. Are the pupils equal and reactive to light?
4. Can the patient move all extremities on command?
5. Are the hand grasps equal and normal in strength?
6. Is the strength of the legs equal and normal?

Neurological assessment should be performed frequently and any changes should be reported to the base station immediately.

Trauma

Head Injury

Head injuries such as fractures, concussions, or contusions may or may not be critical. The patient with major head trauma who is not compensating requires maintenance of ABCs and protection of the spinal cord; then immediate transport with IV and supportive measures instituted enroute. Field treatment of less severe head injuries includes airway management with protection of the spinal column, high-flow oxygen, IV TKO, and frequent reassessment of patient status. If indicated, diuretics and/or steroids might be ordered. Do not give analgesics to a patient with head trauma. All patients with facial or head trauma should be suspected of having had a neck injury and should be securely immobilized before being moved.

Injury to the Spinal Cord

Spinal cord injuries can occur in conjunction with trauma to the face, head, or spinal column, or as a direct result of a penetrating wound. Signs and symptoms may include neck pain, paralysis, decreased sensation, or deformity. Initial treatment consists of airway and respiratory support while protecting the spinal cord. Start an IV TKO and institute supportive measures depending on the severity and extent of the injury. Be prepared to assist ventilations in all patients with cervical spine injuries, as respiratory arrest can occur. Prior to any movement, immobilize the head, neck, and spine. The possibility of spinal cord injury cannot be eliminated based solely on the absence of pain or the ability to move the neck.

Peripheral Nerve Damage

Peripheral nerve damage is usually the result of direct trauma such as burns, falls, or lacerations. Signs and symptoms include pain, paresthesia, or paralysis. Field treatment is primarily supportive and proper splinting techniques should be used to prevent further nerve damage. These types of injuries are rarely a direct threat to life.

Disorders

Coma

Coma is a common field emergency. There are many causes for coma, or depressed brain function, some of these include alcohol, epilepsy, diabetes, shock, overdose, metabolic disorders, trauma, infection, poisoning, stroke, and myocardial infarction. Field treatment includes supportive measures such as airway management, oxygen, monitoring, an IV TKO, intravenous fluids when indicated, stabilization of possible fractures, and diagnostic tools such as Narcan and $D_{50}W$.

Seizures

A wide variety of medical disorders can cause seizures. These include epilepsy, hypoglycemia, hypoxia, arrhythmias, poisoning, hyperthermia, and neurological injury. The significance of a seizure is determined by the situation in which it occurs and the type and length of the seizure activity. Cerebral oxygenation is of primary importance for these patients. Field management consists of maintaining an airway and protecting the patient from injury. High-flow oxygen should be administered immediately following the seizure. In the immediate postictal state, the patient often appears lethargic, somnolent, or disoriented, and may yawn frequently. An IV D_5W TKO may be ordered, and Valium may be required if there are continuous or recurrent seizures, since oxygenation can be impaired during these states. In seizures of unknown etiology, $D_{50}W$ may be given as a diagnostic maneuver. Relay an accurate description of the seizure activity whenever possible as this may help determine the significance of the episode.

Chronic Neurological Disorders

Some patients have chronic neurological disorders which might have acute episodes with potential threat to life. A good history can help disclose the underlying problem and the status of the patient prior to the episode. Some of these chronic disorders include myasthenia gravis, multiple sclerosis, Parkinson's disease, and cerebral palsy. Treatment of these conditions is symptomatic and supportive.

OBSTETRICAL AND GYNECOLOGICAL EMERGENCIES

Childbirth

One of the most important decisions to be made about childbirth in the field is whether there is sufficient time to transport before the infant delivers. Signs of imminent delivery include 1) regular contractions at 1- to 2-minute intervals lasting 45–60 seconds each; 2) a large amount of bloody show; 3) a feeling by the mother of having to bear down or have a bowel movement; 4) crowning, or 5) the mother stating that the baby is coming. If the contractions are short, infrequent, and at irregular intervals, there is probably time to transport.

Normal Childbirth

Field Management of Delivery. Once the decision is made to deliver the infant at the scene, try to provide a sterile field. Wear sterile gloves and prep the perineum with Betadine or saline to help keep the delivery clean. Instruct the mother to bear down only during contractions, and to rest in between to conserve her energy. Guide the infant's head to prevent sudden popping out, which can cause lacerations of the perineum. *Never* forcibly hold the head back to prevent it from delivering. Once the head has delivered, suction the infant's nose and mouth immediately.

Occasionally you will find the umbilical cord wrapped around the baby's neck. This is dangerous because the cord can become too tight and strangle the infant. The cord is usually loose enough for you to slip a couple of fingers around it and lift it over the infant's head. If this is impossible, clamping and cutting the cord before the baby is fully delivered may be the only solution.

As the delivery proceeds, the baby will rotate and the shoulders will present. At this point, guide the head downward to facilitate delivery of the upper shoulder and then upward to deliver the bottom shoulder. The rest of the baby is then delivered with ease. A newborn is extremely slippery, so keep a firm grip on him. Once delivered, attend to the immediate needs of the newborn.

After the cord has stopped pulsating clamp it 6–8 inches from the baby at two points 2 inches apart, and cut the cord between the clamps. Within 10–15 minutes after birth, the placenta should deliver. Suspect that the placenta has separated and its delivery is imminent when you see additional length of cord extending from the vagina in association with a sudden gush of blood.

Save the placenta in a container and take it to the hospital. If difficulty arises with delivery of the placenta, do not pull on the cord or reach into the vagina to try to remove it. It is not necessary for the placenta to deliver prior to transport. Transport mother and infant as soon as possible. Anticipate an IV order for RL or NS. Pitocin may be ordered post delivery to control excessive bleeding, but should never be given in the field before delivery of the placenta.

Ob/Gyn Emergencies

Complications in Childbirth

Prolapsed cord occurs when the cord presents first in the birth canal. Then, with the force of each contraction, it is compressed by the first presenting part of the infant's body, thereby cutting off circulation to the infant. This is a true emergency, for if not corrected, the infant can die. Place the mother in Trendelenberg position with her hips elevated on a pillow. Don't attempt to push the cord back into the vagina. Insert a gloved hand into the vagina and gently manipulate the presenting part so that it no longer compresses the cord. Transport immediately, maintaining this position constantly enroute and until relieved by medical personnel at the hospital. Administer high-flow oxygen and watch for signs of fetal distress, including a drop in fetal heart rate (determined by counting pulsations of the cord) and meconium-stained amniotic fluid. If these signs occur, note the time and report it to the hospital.

Breech deliveries can be readily identified because a foot or buttock presents first as the infant comes out of the birth canal. Most breech deliveries are slow, so you may have time to transport. However, if you are required to deliver an infant in breech presentation, allow the birth to proceed passively until the child is delivered to the waist. Once this occurs, don't pull but gently rotate the baby to a face-down position so that the infant's back is against the mother's pubis. As the delivery proceeds, gently support the limbs by wrapping them in a towel. This will make the baby easier to hold, help keep him warm, and help prevent fractures. If, after 4–6 minutes, the head does not deliver, insert a gloved hand into the vagina and create an airway over the baby's face by forming a V with your index and middle fingers. While maintaining the infant's airway, instruct the mother to bear down and apply *gentle* traction on the upper torso of the infant to facilitate delivery of the head. If you are still unable to deliver the head, transport immediately while maintaining the baby's airway.

Multiple births are an unlikely but possible field occurrence. You must consider this possibility and stay with the mother following delivery of the first infant. Subsequent deliveries can take anywhere from a few minutes to several hours. Each delivery should proceed normally, but there is a higher incidence of difficulty with each delivery, so every effort should be made to transport the mother between births. Once the infant is delivered and the cord is clamped, it is not necessary to cut the cord until all subsequent infants are delivered. Very often, the infants in a multiple birth are premature or unusually small, and one or more may require resuscitation. Watch

44

the mother closely as postpartum hemorrhage is common after multiple births because the uterine muscle has been stretched excessively.

Care of the Newborn

Following birth, the infant should be suctioned vigorously and stimulated to cry. This can be done by slapping the bottoms of his feet or rubbing his back. Determine an Apgar score immediately, and again in 5 minutes using Table 1.2.

Table 1.2. Determining the APGAR Score.

Criteria	Score		
	0	1	2
Color	blue; pale	body pink; extremities blue	all pink
Heart rate	absent	less than 100	greater than 100
Respirations	absent	irregular, slow	good, crying
Reflex response to nose catheter	none	grimace	sneeze, cough
Muscle tone	limp	some reflex of extremities	active

Resuscitate the baby if needed. Monitor respirations closely since newborns, especially premature or small infants, need to be stimulated to continue breathing. If resuscitation is required, use mouth-to-mouth breathing, taking oxygen into your mouth before breathing it into the infant. It is essential to keep the baby warm. Watch the infant closely enroute and let the hospital know you're coming so they can prepare for your arrival.

Complications of Pregnancy

Postpartum Hemorrhage

Postpartum hemorrhage is excessive vaginal bleeding following delivery of an infant. It can be caused by lack of uterine tone, lacerations, or a coagulation defect. Field treatment is aimed at stimulating the uterus to contract. This can be accomplished by massaging the fundus, putting the baby to breast, and/or adding Pitocin to the IV. Additionally, administer high-flow oxygen and monitor patient closely. Transport promptly.

Toxemia of Pregnancy

Seizures during pregnancy are usually a sign of toxemia, a disease which occurs only during pregnancy, and usually in the last trimester. The early stage of toxemia is called pre-eclampsia, and is characterized by high blood pressure, nervousness, malaise, edema, and protein in the urine. In the field, you will probably only see the late stage, eclampsia, which is manifested by seizures and coma. Field treatment of eclampsia is essentially the same as treatment of any other type of seizure, except that care must be taken to protect the fetus as well as the mother. In addition to managing the airway and protecting the patient from injury, you should give high-flow oxygen when the seizure stops. The use of Valium should be reserved only for extreme cases of recurrent or prolonged seizures, as this drug will produce a potentially harmful depressant effect on the fetus. Transport any pregnant seizure patient quickly and maintain a quiet environment, since undue stimuli can precipitate additional seizure activity.

Vaginal Bleeding

Vaginal bleeding during pregnancy can be caused by a variety of disorders, but is usually attributable to one of the following:

Abruptio placenta	placenta separates prematurely from the wall of the uterus
Placenta previa	placenta develops over all or part of the internal cervical opening
Ectopic pregnancy	ovum implants and grows outside the uterus in either the fallopian tube, the ovary, or the abdomen
Spontaneous abortion	pregnancy terminates before the twentieth week of gestation

In the nonpregnant woman, vaginal bleeding is most often caused by menstrual irregularities or problems with an undiagnosed pregnancy. Pelvic inflammatory disease (PID) is a bacterial infection of the female reproductive organs or pelvic cavity which can produce spotting, but more commonly presents with abdominal pain and fever.

The amount of vaginal bleeding depends on the specific causative disorder and its degree of severity. In addition to vaginal bleeding, the patient may have some abdominal pain or cramping, fever, or obvious signs of shock. Regardless of the cause of the bleeding, field treatment is symptomatic and correlated to the severity of the patient's condition. Standard measures would include oxygen, IV (RL or NS) to maintain blood pressure, and prompt transport. Rarely, you may be required to institute extreme shock measures, including antishock trousers and dopamine or vasopressors. No attempt should be made to pack the vagina; this will not control the hemorrhage and may cause harm.

Rape

The rape victim has suffered physical, emotional, and sexual trauma, and may require medical treatment. Although medical management of the patient is vital, emotional support is also critical to the long term psychological survival of the patient. To preserve evidence, minimal treatment should be administered at the scene. Other than control of bleeding and possibly an IV (RL or NS), the appropriate management is close monitoring and prompt transport. Do not attempt to clean the genital area, and don't allow the patient to bathe herself. Collect soiled garments and bring them with you to the ED. Careful observation of the scene and the patient can reveal important information for law enforcement officials.

OVERDOSE

The overdose patient may be found in any one of several stages of distress ranging from asymptomatic or mildly affected to completely apneic, with or without cardiac arrest. The sequence of patient assessment does not change, although you may need to work more quickly due to the urgency of the situation.

Drug overdoses can be caused by prescribed drugs, street drugs, or over-the-counter drugs, alone or in combination, and with or without the associated ingestion of alcohol. The severity of the patient's condition will depend on the type of agent(s), amount ingested, time since ingestion, occurrence of aspiration, preexisting medical conditions, and patient's age. People may overdose themselves deliberately because of job problems, marital discord, or loss of a cherished person or object, or they may overdose accidentally because of improper labeling of the container, poor vision, inadequate lighting, confusion regarding prescribed dosage, or by forgetting how much has already been taken. Regardless of how it occurred, the patient must be assessed and managed without delay.

Field Management of Overdose Patients

Initial assessment includes the ABCs and a determination of level of consciousness. Check for associated injuries, especially fractures or burns, that can accompany overdose. Gather as much information as you can from the patient, the bystanders, and the environment to identify the substance(s) used. If the patient is *unconscious,* check pupil responses, vital signs, lung sounds, and EKG. It is essential to support the airway by proper positioning and the use of airway adjuncts. These patients often vomit, so have suction ready. Assisted ventilation may be required; use an esophageal airway or endo-tracheal tube if the patient is apneic. However, an esophageal airway would be contraindicated when Narcan administration is expected to revive the patient rapidly.

Give high-flow oxygen, start an IV of D_5W TKO, and give Narcan. If the IV can't be established, the Narcan can be injected intra-muscularly, or under the tongue, if the patient is not perfusing. If the sublingual route is used, be sure to control any subsequent bleeding. Narcan might have to be given as many as 10–15 times to be effective. It has a shorter duration of action than the narcotics it inhibits, and thus the patient may again succumb to the effects of the narcotic as the Narcan wears off. For this reason, it is imperative that these patients be transported to the hospital and observed closely for several hours.

Narcan is only effective in reversing the effects of narcotics and opiate derivatives; it is not effective against other sedative agents, e.g. barbiturates. However, it is administered to any unconscious overdose patient because often a combination of drugs which may include a narcotic, has been taken and the patient may be helped by this narcotic antagonist. Narcan is rapid acting and will elicit an immediate response. Very often a patient will become combative following its administration, so protect the IV line from dis-connection. $D_{50}W$ can also be tried in unconscious patients as a diagnostic measure. If the patient has been apneic, sodium bicarbonate may be necessary.

If the patient is *conscious,* get a thorough history of the incident, including the type of agent, amount taken, and time of ingestion. Take vital signs, listen to lung sounds, and monitor EKG. If the induction of vomiting is indicated, and the patient has a gag reflex, you might consider the administration of Syrup of Ipecac. This drug should not be given if the patient ingested an unknown substance or if the substance is known to be caustic or a petroleum distillate. Other contraindications to the use of Syrup of Ipecac include drowsiness, or a decreasing level of consciousness. If none of these contraindications exist, administer Syrup of Ipecac and follow it with large amounts of water. Position the patient to prevent aspiration, and provide a receptacle for the emesis.

Be honest, gentle, and nonjudgmental in your handling of the overdose patient. Explain the importance of proper medical evaluation and management. Protect the airway closely during transport. If the patient has received Syrup of Ipecac, allow him to remain upright in the ambulance to avoid aspiration. Take all medication bottles and drugs with you to the hospital, as well as an emesis sample if the patient vomited.

PEDIATRIC EMERGENCIES

The most competent paramedic is often flustered by a relatively simple problem when it happens to a child. This can be attributed to the fact that children are much more labile than adults, and tend to experience sudden changes in clinical status more readily than adults do. Pediatric patients will be easier to manage if you remember their similarities to and differences from adults.

Most emergencies that happen to an adult can also happen to a child. However, there are certain conditions which occur more often in children; thus, they warrant special discussion in this section. There are disorders that are common in children, such as asthma, diabetes, and poisoning, but which have field treatment that does not differ significantly from that of an adult. These topics are covered in other sections; therefore, they will not be repeated here. Clinical topics specific to children are discussed in later paragraphs.

Approach to Assessment

Your approach to a child in an emergency should be as gentle and nonthreatening as possible. Explain what you are trying to do and what you expect of them. In most cases, it is wise to have a parent present. You might leave a small child in his mother's arms, whereas an older child may be asked to participate in his own care as the situation allows.

Determining Vital Signs

Pediatric vital signs vary from those of adults in that blood pressures are generally lower and pulses and respirations are generally higher. When taking a blood pressure on a child, be sure to use a pediatric cuff; the flush method may be used when auscultation is impractical. The following table approximates pediatric vital signs.

Table 1.3. Vital Signs for Children.

Age	Systolic B/P	Pulse	Respirations
Newborn	50	120	40–60
Child	70–90	95–110	20–30
10–15 year old	110–120	75–85	18–22

Body temperature in a child is also quite different from that of an adult, not in the actual reading but in the fact that it fluctuates so easily. This is why newborns are vulnerable to hypothermia and children frequently have febrile convulsions.

Estimating Pediatric Weights

Because pediatric drug dosages are calculated on the basis of body weight, it is important to remember general guidelines for estimating a child's weight in the field. The information in Table 1.4 refers to *average* children, and requires that you add or subtract weight depending on body build as well as age.

Table 1.4. Average Weight for Children by Age Group.

Age	Weight
newborn	7 pounds
6–12 months	15–22 pounds
2–9 years	add 5 pounds for each year
9–11 years	60–75 pounds

Defibrillation

When defibrillating a child, use pediatric paddles if you can. If this is not possible, use the anterior-posterior paddle placement. The w/s is based on weight; therefore it will be lower for a child than an adult. Current Advanced Cardiac Life Support standards recommend that the w/s setting be calculated using the formula of 3.5–6 w/s per kg. On patients over 50 kg in weight, use the full output of the defibrillator.

Ventilating the Pediatric Patient

The best method of ventilating a child is basic mouth-to-mouth resuscitation. Pediatric Ambu bags and demand valves can be used, but great caution must be exercised to prevent overinflation of the lungs. If endotracheal intubation is necessary, it is essential to select the proper tube size. It is recommended that the endotracheal tube be the size of the patient's little finger.

The Pediatric IV

It takes very little fluid loss to cause hypovolemic shock in a child. Likewise, a relatively small amount of IV fluid replacement can cause overload. For this reason, all pediatric IVs must be set up with a volume control chamber, such as a Volutrol, to avoid inadvertent overload. A safe rate of administration for IV fluid replacement in a hypovolemic child is 20–25 ml/kg/hr.

Field Management of Pediatric Disorders

Upper Airway Obstruction

Upper airway obstruction by foreign objects presents a common problem with children because they enjoy poking small objects into their noses and mouths. When an object occludes the airway you will see signs of obstruction, including respiratory stridor, anxiety, use of accessory muscles of respiration, sternal notch retraction, and cyanosis. Position the child on the side or face down over your arm and try to clear the airway using the finger probe technique. If unsuccesssful, administer four back blows and repeat the cycle. The American Heart Association does not recommend chest thrusts for infants or small children. If total obstruction persists, you may need to look into the airway and remove the object with the Magill forceps, or you may have to consider cricothyrotomy. Following stabilization, give high-flow oxygen and transport to the hospital.

Other disorders which present symptoms similar to airway obstruction are *croup* and *epiglottitis*. These disorders are very similar clinically and are often difficult to differentiate in the field. *Croup* is caused by a virus which results in edema of the subglottic tissues. The patient can exhibit inspiratory stridor, barking cough, dyspnea, and (rarely) cyanosis. This is usually not a severe problem, and it very rarely progresses to total airway obstruction. *Epiglottitis* occurs when a bacterial infection causes the epiglottis to become inflamed. It is extremely dangerous because it can rapidly cause total occulsion of the airway. The symptoms come on suddenly and can include inspiratory stridor, dysphagia, drooling, a high fever, and extreme anxiety. The chin is often thrust forward in a characteristic posture to improve air exchange. Field treatment for both croup and epiglottitis is primarily supportive, including airway maintenance, high-flow oxygen, and prompt transport. It is extremely important to avoid attempts to visualize the epiglottis since this stimulation can cause total obstruction of the airway if epiglottitis is present. Should the airway become completely obstructed, you should try to ventilate, insert an endotracheal tube, or if necessary, perform a cricothyrotomy.

Febrile Convulsions

Febrile convulsions occur when an infection in an infant or child causes the temperature to rise suddenly. This happens because the temperature control center in the brain is immature and allows the temperature to fluctuate unnaturally. Field treatment includes airway management and removal of clothing or heavy bedding. Use cooling measures cautiously; do not use ice or cold water baths. Febrile seizures are usually short in duration, and will often be over by the time you arrive. If the seizures are prolonged or recurrent, IV Valium may be ordered; however, extended seizure activity should suggest something other than febrile convulsions. If accompanied by a stiff neck, seizures might be indicative of meningitis or encephalitis. All patients with seizures should be transported promptly for medical evaluation.

Dehydration

Dehydration can occur quickly in infants and small children following episodes of high fever, vomiting, diarrhea, burns, or excessive urination. With severe depletion of water and electrolytes, a child can show dry mouth, poor skin turgor, weight loss, concentrated or foul-smelling urine, thick secretions, dull vacant-looking eyes, and, in the infant, depressed fontanels. Field treatment includes administration of IV (RL or NS) and supportive measures.

Child Abuse

Child abuse should be suspected in those children who have a personal or sibling history of frequent injuries, particularly when the circumstances don't fit the extent of the injury. Signs suggestive of child abuse include multiple bruises in various healing stages, cigarette or other burns, belt marks, or injuries which are blamed on other people, especially siblings. Treatment is supportive and aimed at managing the presenting problem. Control the ABCs, start an IV if necessary, and bandage or splint wounds appropriately. Be nonjudgmental in your dealings with the parents. Avoid arousing suspicion, as the parents may refuse to allow transport. Report all suspected cases of child abuse to the ED physician so that he can take follow-up action.

Sudden Infant Death Syndrome (SIDS)

Sudden Infant Death Syndrome (SIDS) is a tragic phenomenon, the cause of which remains unknown. Also called "crib death," this syndrome presents a characteristic history of infants who are found dead in their crib without apparent cause. This most commonly strikes children between the ages of one month and one year. Normally, resuscitation attempts will be unsuccessful, but it will comfort the parents to know that every effort was made to help the child. The parents need strong support, as their feelings of guilt and loss are tremendous. Never do or say anything that would suggest parental neglect or responsibility for the death.

POISONING﹡

Poisoning is a very common field emergency that occurs in children 90% of the time. There are countless substances which have been known to cause poisoning in children, e.g., household cleaning products, plants, vitamins and minerals, aspirin, antihistamines and cold medicines. Accidental poisoning in adults is usually caused by carbon monoxide gas, pesticides, chemicals, or drugs. Most adults

---

* The information contained in this section was supplied by the San Diego Regional Poison Information Center, San Diego, California, and relates specifically to prehopsital advanced life support care.

Field Treatment for Poisoning: Unconscious Patient✷

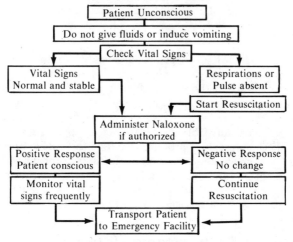

Figure 1.2

Field Treatment for Poisoning: Conscious Patient✷

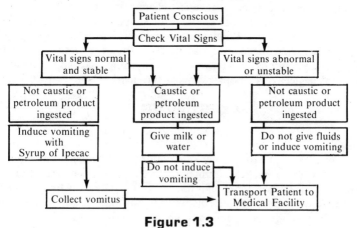

Figure 1.3

✷ Reprinted with permission from *The Journal of Emergency Services*, Carlsbad, California.

who poison themselves intentionally, do so with drugs or carbon monoxide. General guidelines for field management of poisoning in an unconscious and conscious patient are listed in Figures 1.2 and 1.3 respectively.

The paramedic's primary responsibilities in suspected poisoning are to:

1. ensure ABCs, establish level of consciousness and check vital signs
2. support vital functions as needed
3. determine the general nature of the poisonous agent
4. take action to impede absorption of the substance
5. transport promptly

Ingested Substances

For patients who have ingested a poisonous substance, you must first evaluate level of consciousness and resuscitate them if necessary. If the poisonous agent is known to be caustic or is a petroleum distillate, great care must be taken to prevent vomiting, which could create additional damage to the esophagus and oropharynx, or could cause pulmonary complications if aspiration occurs. Do not give anything to induce vomiting. Have the patient drink 6–8 oz. of milk, or water if milk is not available. Do not attempt to insert a nasogastric tube, as this can stimulate the gag reflex or could perforate a weakened esophagus. Give oxygen and transport as rapidly as possible.

If the agent is known to be noncaustic and not a petroleum distillate, and if the patient is alert and has a gag reflex, you can induce vomiting with Syrup of Ipecac. Take care to protect the airway, and allow the patient to remain upright enroute to the hospital. Do not give Syrup of Ipecac if the patient is becoming drowsy.

Differential diagnosis of ingested substances can be time consuming or even impossible in the field, and relates to field treatment only on a superficial level. Specific field treatment will be instituted according to Table 1.5.

Table 1.5.
Field treatment for ingested poisons.

Condition of patient	Agent ingested	Field treatment
• Conscious; has a gag reflex; has stable vital signs	• Known to be non-caustic and not a petroleum distillate	• Give Ipecac; give 6–8 oz. of water or clear beverage; protect airway; transport in an upright position
• Conscious; has a gag reflex; has stable vital signs	• Caustic agent • Petroleum distillate	• Do *not* induce vomiting; give 6–8 oz. milk (preferrably) or water; watch airway closely; give high flow oxygen; transport immediately
• Unconscious • Conscious with unstable vital signs; • Conscious without a gag reflex • Conscious but drowsy	• Narcotic, i.e., codeine, MS, demerol, heroine, paragoric, dilaudid, methadone, lomotil, percodan, darvon; • Unknown agent	• Do *not* induce vomiting; resuscitate if needed; protect airway, give oxygen; monitor EKG; start IV TKO; give Narcan; transport as soon as possible
• Unconscious; • Conscious with unstable vital signs • Conscious without gag reflex • Conscious but drowsy	• Nonnarcotic	• Do *not* induce vomiting; resuscitate if needed; protect airway; give oxygen; monitor EKG and respiratory status; start IV TKO; transport as soon as possible

Toxic Exposure via the Skin

The patient's environment will often identify the causative agent in toxic exposures. As soon as a problem of this nature is suspected, protect yourself from exposure. This would include wearing gloves and keeping the agent away from your clothes and body as much as possible. Quickly remove the patient from the toxic environment. Remove his clothing and wash him down with water to remove chemicals. If you have it available, use soap to clean the chemicals off. Evaluate the vital signs and EKG, and support vital functions as necessary. It may be necessary to delay decontamination until the patient can be stabilized. If the agent is known to be an organophosphate insecticide, start an IV and administer atropine to reverse the parasympathetic effects of the agent. Transport as quickly as possible; monitor EKG and vital signs frequently enroute.

Toxic Inhalations

Protect yourself from the environment and move the patient to fresh air as soon as possible. Give high-flow oxygen and support respirations as needed. Monitor EKG, start an IV TKO, and watch closely enroute.

Home Remedies

Many home remedies and first aid cures have been taught on a large scale, but most have no documented medical value. In fact, they can be very dangerous, and some have been known to cause unnecessary deaths. Some of these "accepted" treatments for poisoning include emetics such as mustard powder, raw eggs, or water to which table salt has been added. These remedies often fail to induce vomiting, and they can be detrimental to the patient or even cause death in some instances.

The universal antidote is a widely recognized remedy which has been shown to be ineffective. Another dangerous treatment commonly recommended is vinegar or citric acid to neutralize ingested alkalis such as drain cleaners. This does neutralize the agent, but in the process it generates an intense heat that is severe enough to produce thermal burns of the oropharynx and esophagus, thereby complicating the original injury. These procedures are dangerous and should never be practiced in the field. If you have a regional Poison

Information Center, you or the base hospital can contact them to obtain additional information for emergency treatment.

General

Always try to bring with you to the hospital any containers or clues from the scene that will help the laboratory identify the toxic agent. If the patient vomits, bring a sample of the emesis to the hospital for analysis. The primary concern of the paramedic is to avoid causing further harm to the patient during the treatment process. Monitor the patient closely, especially respiratory status, and transport as quickly as possible.

RESPIRATORY EMERGENCIES

The upper respiratory tract is comprised of the nose, mouth, oropharynx, larynx, and trachea and serves specifically to filter, humidify, and warm inspired air. The lower respiratory tract consists of the mainstem bronchi, bronchioles, and terminal air sacs (alveoli). It is in the alveoli that gaseous exchange takes place, i.e., the elimination of carbon dioxide and the uptake of oxygen. Interruption of this vital system along any of its structures can result in respiratory distress and subsequent death. Some of the more common disorders that can disrupt the normal respiratory process are discussed in the following paragraphs.

Common Respiratory Disorders

Asthma

Asthma can be caused by allergic hypersensitivity reaction to a foreign substance, e.g., pollen, smog, or food, or it can be brought on by psychological stress. Asthma is manifested by bronchial constriction and an increase in thick mucus production resulting in decreased oxygen exchange. Signs and symptoms include dyspnea, restlessness, apprehension, prolonged expiratory phase, wheezing, tachycardia, and varying degrees of hypoxia. Treatment includes humidified high-flow oxygen, hydration to reduce viscosity and allow expulsion of mucous plugs, and reassurance. Additionally, bronchial constriction can be reduced with bronchodilators such as Isuprel Mistometer, Epinephrine, or Aminophylline.

Chronic Bronchitis

Chronic Bronchitis is an inflammation of the bronchial tree which results in abundant mucus production and a chronic cough. This disorder can be caused by pollution, dust, fumes, cigarette smoke, and viral or bacterial agents. Signs and symptoms include a productive cough (usually without fever), dyspnea, wheezes, rhonchi, a prolonged expiratory phase, and cyanosis in the late stages. The bronchitic patient is usually stocky in stature and may have associated congestive heart failure due to chronic pulmonary congestion. Treatment of acute episodes is supportive, consisting of *low*-flow oxygen, position of comfort, and reassurance. You may need to administer Aminophylline for severe respiratory distress.

Emphysema

Emphysema is caused by loss of elasticity within the alveoli, resulting in enlargement of the terminal air sacs. This loss of elasticity causes the smaller airways to collapse on expiration, thus trapping air in the alveoli and resulting in hypoxemia. The patient breathes through pursed lips in an unconscious effort to prevent collapse of the alveoli. Other signs and symptoms of advanced emphysema include emaciation, fatigue, barrel chest, use of accessory muscles for respiration, prolonged expiratory phase, and cyanosis. Field treatment of acute episodes consists primarily of *low*-flow oxygen. Transport in a position of comfort – usually sitting up and forward – and be supportive. You may need to administer Aminophylline for severe respiratory distress.

Chronic Obstructive Pulmonary Disease

Chronic obstructive pulmonary disease (COPD) is a general phrase referring to any longstanding respiratory disorder which results in obstruction of gaseous exchange in the alveoli. It most commonly encompasses emphysema and bronchitis, but also can be used to describe other chronic respiratory diseases as well. In a healthy person, the respiratory drive comes from a high serum carbon dioxide level, whereas the COPD patient requires a low serum oxygen level for respiratory stimulus. For this reason, the administration of high-flow oxygen can be detrimental to the COPD patient as it can cause loss of the respiratory drive with resultant apnea.

COPD is a prevalent condition, and is often a complicating factor in patients who seek emergency help for unrelated medical conditions. Patients experiencing acute medical emergencies often require oxygen to manage their immediate illness. If the patient has underlying COPD, the oxygen should be started at a low flow rate of 1-2 liters/minute and increased cautiously only if the patient continues to show signs of hypoxia. If an increase in flow rate is needed to manage the immediate situation, be prepared to support respirations if the patient's own respiratory drive is lost.

Pulmonary Embolus

Pulmonary embolism occurs when a blood clot travels from one part of the body and lodges in a pulmonary blood vessel, occluding circulation to a portion of the lungs. Predisposing factors to pulmonary emboli include inactivity, recent surgery, pregnancy, varicose veins, or use of birth control pills. Signs and symptoms are dependent on the amount of tissue damage, but can include pleuritic chest pain of sudden onset, dyspnea, diaphoresis, hemoptysis, fever, cyanosis, and profound shock in severe cases. Treatment consists of high-flow oxygen, an IV of D_5W TKO, symptomatic life support, and prompt transport.

Pleurisy

Pleurisy is an inflammation of the lining of the lung causing localized pain on inspiration due to the pleura rubbing against each other. Respirations are usually rapid and shallow as the patient attempts to splint his breathing and reduce the pain. Once again, treatment consists of high-flow oxygen, an IV of D_5W TKO, and supportive care.

Pneumonia

Pneumonia is an inflammatory process involving the alveoli. It may be caused by bacteria, virus, or aspiration. Signs and symptoms include fever, cough with large amounts of dark-colored sputum, chest pain on inspiration, flushed face, weak and rapid pulse, and dyspnea. In advanced cases, rales, rhonchi, and areas of decreased breath sounds can be heard on auscultation. Field treatment is limited, but might include oxygen, an IV of D_5W TKO, close monitoring, and support of respirations.

Spontaneous Pneumothorax

Spontaneous pneumothorax is a partially or totally collapsed lung, the result of a ruptured bleb on the pleural lining. It occurs without warning and most commonly strikes young adult males. It can frequently be identified by sudden onset of dyspnea, cough, and a sharp pain which might be referred to the shoulder. Breath sounds can be diminished or absent on the affected side. Field treatment is supportive, and may include ventilatory assistance, an IV of D_5W TKO, and monitoring of EKG.

Smoke/Gas Inhalation

The inhalation of noxious substances such as smoke or toxic gases create a medical emergency by one or more of the following mechanisms:

- Asphyxiation: Oxygen exchange is prevented
- Irritation: The substance itself causes damage to the lung tissue
- Poisoning: The inhaled agent introduces a poisonous substance into the blood stream via the lungs

Patients with inhalation injury can often be recognized when their chief complaint is respiratory difficulty and they are located near the source of a gas, such as a chemical plant, a heater, or a fire. They may experience cough, pain on inspiration, depressed level of consciousness, seizures, or rigidity. Patients with carbon monoxide poisoning, for example, often complain only of a throbbing headache coincidental with unusual giddiness.

Although specific treatments have been developed for certain distinct gases, field treatment for all inhalation injuries remains basic. Immediately remove the patient from the gas source and support respirations while giving high-flow oxygen. It may be necessary to ventilate with positive pressure, and the patient should be monitored closely. Some inhaled irritants result in laryngeal edema, so advanced airway techniques such as endotracheal intubation or cricothyrotomy may be indicated. Do not administer any analgesics, as respiratory depression can develop. An IV of D_5W TKO may be ordered. Monitor EKG and transport promptly.

SHOCK

Shock can be defined as perfusion which is inadequate to maintain cellular metabolsim, thus resulting in cellular anoxia and tissue death. The problem may be caused by decreased circulating volume due to loss of blood or fluid, decreased efficiency of the heart as a pump, or generalized vasodilatation. In all cases, a cycle develops which must be interrupted before it becomes irreversible.

There are several different kinds of shock and an accurate identification is necessary in order to select the appropriate therapy.

Hypovolemic Shock

Hypovolemic shock is caused by inadequate circulating blood volume, and may be precipitated by severe traumatic or gastrointestinal bleeding, or fluid loss following extensive diarrhea, vomiting, or burns. Signs and symptoms include restlessness, anxiety, mental sluggishness, cool clammy skin, pallor, tachycardia, rapid shallow respirations, thirst, and *possibly* hypotension. Field treatment consists of hemorrhage control, oxygen, elevation of the lower extremities (if not contraindicated), volume replacement with RL or NS and rarely saltpoor albumin (SPA). If indicated, apply antishock trousers in severe cases. If fluid replacement and the antishock trousers fail, dopamine or vasopressors may be needed to support the cardiovascular system.

Cardiogenic Shock

Cardiogenic shock is caused by inefficient pumping action of the heart, and can follow a massive MI, sustained tachyarrhythmias, acute valvular insufficiency, pericardial tamponade, pulmonary embolus, tension pneumothorax, or end-stage CHF with pulmonary edema. Signs and symptoms are essentially the same as hypovolemic shock except that hypotension is severe. Treatment is aimed at improving tissue oxygenation and increasing the efficiency of the heart as a pump. Field treatment includes high-flow oxygen, an IV of D_5W TKO, dopamine or vasopressors, arrhythmia suppression as needed, and treatment of associated injuries or illnesses. This is a critical condition and warrants very close monitoring of vital signs and EKG and prompt transport.

Low-Resistance Shock

Low-resistance shock, or neurogenic shock, occurs when there is a pathologic disparity between the circulating blood volume and the dilated vascular space, creating a relative blood loss. This can occur in septic shock, spinal cord trauma, certain drug overdoses, anaphylactic shock, or heat stroke. Signs and symptoms depend on the etiology, but are similar to other forms of shock and will usually include a drop in blood pressure. Since generalized vasodilatation has occurred, cool, clammy skin may not be as apparent as with other kinds of shock.

Give high-flow oxygen, monitor EKG, start an IV for possible fluid replacement, elevate the legs if not contraindicated, check for associated injuries or illnesses, and apply antishock trousers if appropriate. Dopamine or vasopressors may be needed to support the cardiovascular system if other antishock measures are not effective. Treatment of low-resistance shock is aimed at the cause of the condition; specific drug therapy may be indicated.

SELF ASSESSMENT QUESTIONS

ASSESSMENT

1. Discuss the importance of effective patient assessment.

2. Discuss the components of primary and secondary surveys.

3. What are the ABCs, and how should they be assessed?

4. What clues are available from the scene and how should they be gathered?

5. What types of patients require immediate transport and why?

6. Define the term "chief complaint" and describe how it can direct your patient assessment.

7. Discuss the history questions you can ask to pursue the chief complaint.

8. Discuss the various components of the vital signs and explain the factors that must be evaluated for each.

9. List four evaluative tools used in performing a physical examination and discuss the field application of each.

10. Describe the head-to-toe field examination.

11. Discuss the importance of accurate reporting of assessment information.

ACUTE ABDOMINAL PAIN

1. What is the most common cause of shock associated with acute abdominal pain?

2. What clinical disorder is suggested when you see a pulsating mass in the abdomen?

3. Why do you *not* palpate a pulsating abdominal mass?

4. Why is prompt transport indicated for patients with acute abdominal pain?

5. List two contraindications in the treatment of patients with acute abdominal pain.

6. What is the clinical picture of a patient with abdominal pain?

7. Discuss general priniciples for treating patients with abdominal pain.

AIRWAY OBSTRUCTION
(Foreign Body)

1. Why is an obstructed airway a true emergency?

2. List five things which commonly obstruct the airway.

3. Why don't you treat patients with an airway obstruction who are able to talk and cough?

4. How would you distinguish a partial airway obstruction from a complete airway obstruction?

5. List the steps in treating a conscious patient with obstructed airway who has ineffective breathing.

6. List the steps necessary to treat an unconscious patient with obstructed airway.

ANAPHYLACTIC SHOCK

1. Discuss the pathophysiology of anaphylaxis:
   a. blood vessels
   b. bronchial tree
   c. cell permeability

2. List the agents commonly responsible for producing anaphylaxis.

3. Relate the signs and symptoms of anaphylaxis to its physiology.

4. Discuss field management of a patient experiencing anaphylactic reaction.

5. Discuss the pharmacological actions of Epinephrine and Benadryl in the treatment of anaphylaxis.

6. In a severe anaphylactic reaction, what additional drug therapy might be indicated?

BEHAVIORAL EMERGENCIES

1. Discuss categories of behavioral emergencies.

2. List medical disorders that can mimic behavioral emergencies and explain the value of differential diagnosis in the field.

3. Discuss the categorization of behavioral emergencies:
   a. acute drug intoxication
   b. acute alcohol intoxication
   c. acute psychiatric disorders
   d. withdrawal syndrome

4. Discuss field management techniques for quiet or suicidal patients and for aggressive patients.

5. Discuss the primary goal in the field management of patients exhibiting aberrant behavior.

6. Discuss local legal considerations in behavioral emergencies, including consent and legal restraint.

BURNS

1. Discuss the pathophysiology of a burn injury.

2. List the signs and symptoms that differentiate first, second, and third degree burns.

3. List three sources of burn injuries.

4. List the signs and symptoms indicative of a respiratory burn.

5. Discuss the "Rule of Nines."

6. How do you calculate percentage of burns in children?

7. List the complications which can occur in a burn injury.

8. List those burns which are considered critical and need to be transported.

9. List the field treatment for:
   a. thermal burns
   b. chemical burns
   c. electrical burns
   d. respiratory burn

10. Discuss the contraindications in burn therapy.

CARDIOGENIC SHOCK

1. Define cardiogenic shock.

2. List possible causes of cardiogenic shock.

3. What signs and symptoms would suggest a patient is in cardiogenic shock?

4. Discuss the field management of cardiogenic shock following an MI.

5. Why are excessive IV fluids contraindicated in cardiogenic shock?

CEREBROVASCULAR ACCIDENT (CVA)

1. Discuss the pathophysiology of CVA.

2. List factors which may contribute to CVA.

3. List the signs and symptoms of CVA.

4. Discuss the field treatment of CVA.

5. Discuss transient ischemic attacks and their significance.

CHEST TRAUMA

1. Discuss the pathophysiology and related signs and symptoms of
   a. traumatic pneumothorax/hemothorax
   b. tension pneumothorax
   c. flail chest
   d. open chest injuries
   e. cardiac trauma

2. Describe field treatment for:
   a. traumatic pneumothorax/hemothorax
   b. tension pneumothorax
   c. flail chest
   d. open chest injuries
   e. cardiac trauma

CONGESTIVE HEART FAILURE (CHF)

1. List conditions which contribute to CHF.

2. Differentiate between the signs and symptoms of left- and right-sided heart failure and relate them to their respective pathophysiologies.

3. List the signs and symptoms of pulmonary edema and relate them to the underlying pathophysiology.

4. List the field treatment of CHF, including the pharmacological agents.

DIABETES

1. Discuss the pathophysiology and related clinical manifestations of diabetes, including the two extremes of hypoglycemia and hyperglycemia.

2. Why is hypoglycemia so dangerous?

3. Discuss clues at the scene and on patients which can help diagnose unconscious patients as diabetics.

4. Discuss field management for patients who are hypoglycemic and:
   a. conscious
   b. unconscious
   c. losing consciousness

5. Discuss field management of diabetic patients who cannot be diagnosed accurately as being hyperglycemic or hypoglycemic, whether they are
   a. conscious
   b. unconscious
   c. losing consciousness

6. Discuss the use of IV fluid replacement in hyperglycemia.

DROWNING

1. What are the two main physiological problems resulting from a near-drowning?

2. List factors that could influence the severity of the problems exhibited by near-drowning patients.

3. Why is a thorough physical examination essential for all neardrowning patients?

4. Discuss the field treatment for a near-drowning patient who is (a) asymptomatic, mildly effected or (b) symptomatic or in full arrest.

5. Why is it important to obtain a specimen of the water in which persons almost drowned?

6. Why is it mandatory to transport all near-drowning victims?

ENVIRONMENTAL EMERGENCIES

1. Differentiate between *local* and *systemic* signs and symptoms of envenomation following a snake bite.

2. Describe proper field treatment of a patient who has been bitten by a venomous snake.

3. Discuss the recognition and field management of stingray injury and jellyfish sting.

4. Discuss recognition and field management of poisonous spider bites.

5. Differentiate between heat exposure, heat exhaustion, and heat stroke, discussing signs and symptoms and field management.

6. Discuss the recognition and field management of general body cooling and frostbite.

7. List signs and symptoms and field management of radiation exposure.

MAJOR TRAUMA AND TRIAGE

1. Describe priorities for patient assessment in multiple-trauma patients.

2. Discuss components to be included in the management of ABCs in multiple-trauma patients.

3. Discuss contraindications of care for multiple-trauma patients.

4. Define triage and explain its use in the field.

5. Describe the categories used in triage — immediate, urgent, minimal, and delayed treatment.

6. Describe the functions of the patient man and the radio man during triage situations.

7. Discuss the criteria you would use for setting priorities of care in multiple patient situations.

8. Discuss the "best for the most" philosophy of triage.

9. Discuss the importance of record-keeping in triage situations.

10. Discuss the factors to be considered when loading ambulances.

MYOCARDIAL INFARCTION (MI)

1. Discuss the pathophysiology of an MI.

2. Describe the pain of an MI.

3. In addition to pain, what other signs and symptoms can be associated with an MI?

4. Discuss the field treatment of an MI.

5. List the three most common complications of an MI.

6. What is the most common cause of death after a patient suffers an MI?

7. Discuss the role arrhythmias play in the course of an MI. Include the most common arrhythmias, their significance and their treatment.

8. Discuss the use of the following drugs in an MI:
   • morphine
   • atropine
   • lidocaine

9. Why are oxygen, an IV, and EKG monitoring mandatory in any suspected MI?

NEUROLOGICAL EMERGENCIES

1. Discuss neurological assessment.

2. Discuss increasing intracranial pressure with respect to causes, signs and symptoms and field management.

3. Discuss the field management of major head trauma (when patients are not compensating) and less severe head injuries.

4. Discuss the importance of noting alterations in level of consciousness following a head injury.

5. Why should patients with head injuries be immobilized?

6. What precaution must be taken in the airway maintenance of patients with head injuries?

7. Discuss the causes of spinal cord trauma.

8. What signs and symptoms would make you suspect a spinal cord injury?

9. Discuss precautionary measures to be taken with suspected or actual spinal cord injury.

10. Discuss the causes, signs and symptoms, and field management of peripheral nerve damage.

11. Give five common conditions that can present with unconsciousness.

12. Discuss common causes of seizures.

13. How is a seizure managed in the field?

14. Discuss the management of recurrent or continuous seizures.

15. Describe the postictal state.

16. List three chronic neurological disorders that may have acute episodes.

OBSTETRICAL AND GYNECOLOGICAL (OB/GYN) EMERGENCIES

1. List the signs indicating an imminent delivery.

2. Describe considerations in normal childbirth:
   a. delivery of the infant
   b. umbilical cord around the baby's neck
   c. delivery of the placenta
   d. care of the newborn

3. Discuss the pathophysiology, signs and symptoms, and field management of:
   a. prolapsed cord
   b. fetal distress
   c. breech deliveries

d. multiple births
e. postpartum hemorrhage
f. maternal seizures
g. vaginal bleeding

4. Describe the APGAR rating scale.

5. Discuss the field management of the rape victim.

OVERDOSE

1. List common substances used in overdosing.

2. What factors determine the severity of overdosed patients?

3. Discuss assessment of overdosed patients.

4. List the field treatment of overdosed patients who are unconscious or conscious.

5. Discuss the use of Narcan for unconscious overdosed patients including the following:
   a. route, indications, and contraindications
   b. alternate routes of administration
   c. need to repeat

6. Discuss the use of Syrup of Ipecac in overdosed patients including indications, contraindications and positioning the patient.

7. Discuss the use of the esophageal airway in overdosed patients.

8. Discuss attitudinal problems encountered in managing overdosed patients.

PEDIATRIC EMERGENCIES

1. Describe techniques which may help ease anxiety and facilitate emergency care in pediatric patients.

2. Discuss vital sign techniques and give normal ranges for:
   • newborn
   • child
   • 10–15 year old

3. How and why are drug dosages calculated for children?

4. Discuss weight approximations according to age.

5. Discuss defibrillation of children; include calculation of w/s setting.

6. Discuss the use of positive pressure ventilators with infants and children.

7. Describe pediatric IV fluid therapy, including amount of solution and precautions with administration.

8. List signs, symptoms, and field management of:
   a. upper airway obstruction
   b. croup/epiglottitis
   c. febrile seizures
   d. dehydration
   e. child abuse
   f. sudden infant death syndrome

POISONING

1. Discuss the agents most commonly involved in:
   a. pediatric poisoning
   b. adult accidental poisoning
   c. adult intentional poisoning

2. List the five primary responsibilities in field care of poisoned patients.

3. Discuss recognition and field management of:
   a. ingested poisons
   b. toxic exposures on the skin
   c. toxic inhalations

4. Discuss common home remedies which can be detrimental to poisoned patients.

5. List clues from the scene of the poisoning which can help the hospital identify toxic substance.

RESPIRATORY EMERGENCIES

1. What are the structures and functions of the respiratory system?

2. Discuss the pathophysiology, signs and symptoms, and field treatment of:

   a. asthma
   b. chronic bronchitis
   c. emphysema
   d. pulmonary embolus
   e. pleurisy
   f. pneumonia
   g. spontaneous pneumothorax
   h. smoke/gas inhalation

3. What precautions should be taken with the use of oxygen on COPD patients, and why should they be taken?

4. What drugs are used to alleviate respiratory distress in the field?

SHOCK

1. Discuss the pathophysiology, signs, and symptoms of hypovolemic, cardiogenic and low-resistance shock.

2. Discuss field management of the three types of shocks in question 1.

3. Why is it important to distinguish which type of shock is present?

TREATMENT PROTOCOLS

INTRODUCTION

The purpose of this section on treatment protocols is to help paramedics visualize the total picture of prehospital advanced life support care. Additionally, familiarity with treatment protocols can help base hospitals to better understand the paramedic's role and field capabilities. These protocols are *not* intended to dictate medical practices but are designed to bring together the important facts about many common emergency conditions into a single source. In this format, these protocols can be modified to conform to local medical practices.

The 32 medical conditions in this section were selected because they are the ones most often encountered by paramedics. Each of the topics is subdivided according to specific treatments, so that the total set should cover most of the emergencies which you can be prepared to manage effectively.

Because emergencies often occur with more than one major problem, such as chest pain with arrhythmias, it might be necessary to use more than one protocol for a single call. However, it is far more effective to use individual rather than combined protocols.

Treatment protocols are designed to be a summary of all the important facts about a particular problem. The information on each protocol should be committed to memory. These summaries are for reference, and are not intended to "walk you through" an emergency situation. For this reason, they must be thoroughly understood *before* you need them, not learned during the emergency. If the base hospital would like to use them as a guide during a call, then each hospital should modify the format to suit its needs. The important thing to remember is that these protocols are intended to be comprehensive. Therefore, they cannot be as concise as they need to be when used as a reference during an emergency.

Accordingly, each protocol attempts to anticipate all of the possible complications that might arise in any given condition. Obviously, not all of these will happen with every run, so much of each protocol will go unused during a particular call. Also, the order of the protocol will very rarely, if ever, be followed strictly as written, since individual patient data will necessitate different responses. It would be inappropriate and highly irresponsible to conduct each run by asking all of the questions in the order listed in these protocols, or to withhold treatment until a complete history is obtained. These protocols are *not* a substitute for your own medical knowledge, experience, and judgment and you should make your own decisions. Remember, too, that these protocols are for prehospital care, and as such are not readily adapted to the inhospital management of emergency patients.

Some disorders will require immediate transport without any delay in the field because the stabilization they require is only available within the hospital. We include in this category all situations where the patient is not tolerating the injury, specifically aneurysms, major head, chest or abdominal trauma, or trauma to more than one system. For these urgent states, the paramedic should transport the patient immediately, contact the hospital and initiate treatment enroute.

The hospital has the ultimate responsibility for directing not only the field treatment rendered by the paramedic, but also the disposition of the patient to an appropriate emergency facility. Since the hospital has the advantage of being able to assess patient condition in the prehospital setting via the paramedic, the patient should be taken directly to the emergency facility that has been designated by the regional Emergency Medical Services (EMS) plan as the most appropriate facility for that specific problem.

ABDOMINAL PAIN
(Nontraumatic)

History

- What type of pain is it?
- Where is the pain located?
- Does the pain radiate?
- When did it start?
- What precipitated it?
- Has the patient ever had it before?
- What is the severity of the pain?
- What is the pain associated with?
- Has the patient had any recent illnesses or operations?
- Did the patient suffer recent trauma?
- Has the patient had any changes in bowel or bladder habits?
- Has the patient been nauseated or vomited?
- Did the patient ingest any unusual substances?
- Has there been any vaginal bleeding or discharge?

Physical Exam

- What is the respiratory status?
- What is the patient's level of consciousness?
- What is the skin color, moisture, and temperature?
- What are the vital signs?
- What is the EKG pattern?
- Are there any signs of dehydration?
- Is the patient febrile?
- Is the patient "guarding"?
- Are there bruises, pulsating masses, or scars on the abdomen?
- Is the abdomen rigid?

Differential Diagnosis

- Can be any variety of medical disorder.
- Needs inhospital work-up.

Treatment

Field management is limited

1. Assure the airway, especially if vomiting has occurred.
2. Give oxygen.
3. Start an IV of D_5W TKO; if hypovolemic shock is suspected, start RL or NS at a rapid rate.
4. An NG tube may be ordered.
5. If blood loss is significant, antishock trousers may be indicated.
6. Do not give analgesics or oral fluids.
7. Do not waste time palpating the abdomen extensively or eliciting bowel sounds.

Special Note

- Save any stool, urine, or emesis and take it to the hospital for analysis.

Pediatric Note

- In a child, suspect poisoning.

Transport

- Patient should be transported as soon as possible.
- Do not delay transportation for diagnostic maneuvers.

ABDOMINAL TRAUMA

History

- Was the trauma blunt or penetrating?
- What was the time of injury?
- When was the onset of symptoms?

- What was the mechanism of injury?
- Where is the injury?
- What type of pain is involved?
- What is the estimated blood loss?

Physical Exam

- What is the respiratory and cardiovascular status?
- What is the patient's level of consciousness?
- What is the skin color, temperature, and moisture?
- What are the vital signs?
- Are there any apparent injuries on front or back?
- Are there any associated injuries?
- Are there any penetrating objects?
- If gunshot or knife injury, are there exit wounds?

Differential Diagnosis

- Perform thorough exam for other injuries.

Treatment

1. Assure the airway, give oxygen, ventilate if necessary.
2. Control bleeding.
3. Start an IV of RL or NS and run at a rapid rate to maintain blood pressure. May need to use a volume expander.
4. If blood loss is significant, antishock trousers may be indicated.
5. Do not give analgesics or oral fluids.
6. Do not waste time palpating the abdomen extensively or eliciting bowel sounds.
7. If the patient has an eviscerated bowel, cover with saline-soaked pads.
8. Immobilize patient before moving, if indicated.

Special Note

- Any high abdominal injury should be suspected of involving the thoracic cavity.
- Penetrating objects should be immobilized but not removed unless antishock trousers need to be applied over them.

Pediatric Note

- Consider child abuse.

Transport

- Transport the patient as soon as possible.

AIRWAY OBSTRUCTION
(Foreign Body)

History

- When did this happen?
- What precipitated the event?
- Was the patient eating or putting things in his mouth?
- Were there any other medical complaints such as chest pain or a bee sting?

Physical Exam

- Is the patient exchanging air effectively?
- What are the sounds of respiration?
- What is the level of consciousness?
- Is the patient able to talk or cough?
- What is the skin color?

Differential Diagnosis

- Must be differentiated from laryngeal edema.

Treatment

(Paramedic does not need an order to proceed as follows)

If the patient is *conscious and able to talk or cough:*
1. Leave him alone.
2. Give reassurance.
3. Encourage him to cough.
4. Give oxygen if he will tolerate it.

If the patient is *conscious but unable to talk or exchange air:*
1. Administer four back blows.
2. Administer four manual thrusts.
3. Repeat steps 1 and 2.

If the patient is *unconscious when found or loses consciousness:*
1. Open airway and attempt to ventilate.
2. Reposition head and attempt to ventilate again.
3. Try to remove foreign body with Magill forceps and laryngoscope.
4. If unsuccessful or if Magill forceps are not immediately available, administer four back blows and four manual thrusts.
5. Repeat steps 2–4; if unsuccessful, transport Code 3 while continuing the series.
6. Consider cricothyrotamy if all other maneuvers fail.

Special Note

- Once obstruction is removed, assess patient for bilateral air movement, color, respiratory effort and vital signs; monitor EKG, give high-flow oxygen, and start an IV of D_5W TKO if necessary.
- All patients in this category must be evaluated at the hospital since part of the obstruction may have remained

in the respiratory tract and will cause infection and/or irritation.

Pediatric Note

- Consider the possibility of croup.
- Children often insert foreign objects into nose or mouth.
- If epiglottitis is suspected, do not attempt to visualize the oropharynx, as the airway may obstruct totally; transport Code 3; if respiratory arrest occurs, ventilate and perform endotracheal intubation or cricothyrotomy.

Transport

- No need for Code 3 if patient is stabilized.

ALLERGIC REACTION

History

- Was the patient recently exposed to foods, drugs, insects, or other allergens that may have induced reaction?
- When was patient exposed?
- When did symptoms appear?
- Has the patient had previous allergic reactions?

Physical Exam

- Are there any signs of respiratory distress or tightness in the chest?
- Are there any signs of systemic allergic reaction such as rash, itching, hives, or general swelling?
- What is the level of consciousness?
- What is the skin color, temperature, and moisture?
- What are the vital signs?
- Are the lungs clear to auscultation?
- What is the EKG pattern?

• Is the patient wearing a Medic-Alert tag?

Differential Diagnosis

• Might be confused with asthma or foreign body obstruction of the upper airway.
• Determine the source of the reaction, such as bee, drug, or food.
• Differentiate between allergic reaction and true anaphylactic shock.

Treatment

1. Give oxygen and ventilate if necessary.
2. Place a constricting band 1 inch proximal to site if feasible.
3. Give Epinephrine 0.3 mg 1:1000 SC may repeat; can also give 0.1 mg 1:1000 at site if other than fingers or toes.
4. Start an IV of D_5W TKO.
5. If laryngeal edema or hypotension is present, give 0.5–1 mg Epinephrine 1:10,000 IV push in 1 ml increments titrated to blood pressure.
6. Give Benadryl 25–50 mg IM or IV push.
7. Keep patient calm, discourage activity.
8. May need additional drug therapy such as Aminophyliine, dopamine, or vasopressors.
9. If cardiovascular collapse continues despite drug therapy, apply antishock trousers.
10. May need cricothyrotomy if patient does not respond to drugs and airway becomes totally obstructed.

Special Note

• If reaction is severe, attempt to intubate before edema occludes the airway.

Pediatric Note

- Should not give aminophylline to children under 12 years of age.
- Pediatric doses:
  Benadryl: 2–5 mg/kg slow IV push or IM
  Epinephrine: 0.1 mg 1:1000 SC, up to 0.3 mg
  Dopamine: 5μg/kg/min IV drip

Transport

- May need epinephrine enroute.
- Need not be Code 3 if patient is stabilized.

ARRHYTHMIAS

History

- Is the patient exhibiting chest pain, palpitations, or shortness of breath?
- When did symptoms begin?
- What precipitated them?
- Has the patient ever had them before?
- Has the patient ever had cardiac problems or arrhythmias before?
- Is the patient taking any medications?

Physical Exam

- Are there any signs or symptoms of decreased cardiac output, such as anxiety, dyspnea, dizziness, substernal chest pain, diaphoresis, pallor, or decreased level of consciousness?
- What are the vital signs?
- Are the lungs clear to auscultation?
- What is the EKG pattern?
- Does the patient have signs of congestive heart failure?

Differential Diagnosis

Drop in cardiac output can be caused by
- Tachycardias
- Bradycardias
- Ventricular arrhythmias.

Treatment

- Treatments will not necessarily be initiated in this order, nor will all drugs/maneuvers listed be given for every rhythm, since arrhythmias with varying severity will require more or less aggressive treatments.
- All patients with arrhythmias (or the potential for them) should receive an IV of D₅W TKO.
- All rhythms that cause respiratory impairment and/or cardiac arrest will require basic resuscitative measures as well as sodium bicarbonate, 1 mEq/kg IV push initially; this dose can be repeated. Thereafter one-half the initial dose can be given at 10 minute intervals.

Tachycardias (including SVT, PAT)
1. Give high-flow oxygen
2. Perform vagotonic maneuvers (Valsalva's, CSM)
3. Give Inderal 0.5 mg IV push every minute for a total of no more than 4 mg, titrate to effect; *or* give Digoxin 0.25–0.5 mg slow IV push
4. Perform synchronized cardioversion; if necessary, sedate patient with Valium in increments of 2.5 mg IV push up to 15 mg. Watch for apnea.

Bradycardias (including supraventricular, heart blocks, idioventricular rhythm, asystole)
1. Give high-flow oxygen
2. Assist ventilations as needed
3. Give atropine sulfate 0.5–1 mg IV push for a total of no more than 2 mg (for

supraventricular bradycardias and heart blocks)

4. Give Isuprel 1–2 mg in 250–500 ml D₅W, titrate to pulse (for heart blocks, idioventricular rhythm, and asystole)
5. Give Epinephrine 0.5–1 mg 1:10,000 IV push (for idioventricular rhythm and asystole)
6. Give calcium chloride 250–500 mg IV push or IC (for electromechanical dissociation or asystole after sodium bicarbonate and Epinephrine are on board)

Ventricular (including tachycardia, ectopics)

1. Give high-flow oxygen
2. If patient is conscious:
   a) Give lidocaine 50–100 mg IV push
   b) give lidocaine 1–2 gm in 250–500 ml D₅W and adjust it to administer no more than 4 mg/kg/hour
3. If patient is unconscious and in ventricular tachycardia, perform synchronized cardioversion or defibrillation using 3.5–6.0 w/s per kg of body weight up to 50 kg; over 50 kg use full output of the defibrillator
4. Following cardioversion or defibrillation administer lidocaine bolus and drip
5. For ventricular ectopics in the presence of a bradycardia, give Atropine 0.5–1 mg IV push

Ventricular (fibrillation)

1. Perform CPR and ventilate
2. If observed, defibrillate
3. If unobserved, administer NaHCO₃ 1 mEq/kg and Epinephrine 0.5-1 mg prior to defibrillation
4. Following conversion, give lidocaine bolus and drip

Special Note

• Cardiac arrhythmias are treated only if they are causing,

or have the potential to cause, symptoms of decreased cardiac output.

Pediatric Note

Pediatric doses:
- Inderal 0.1 mg/kg slow IV push; may repeat in 15 minutes (initial maximum dose is 2 mg).
- Valium 0.05 mg/kg slow IV push.
- Atropine 0.01–0.02 mg/kg IV push.
- Isuprel 1 mg in 250–500 ml D_5W; titrate to pulse.
- Epinephrine 1:10,000; 0.1 ml/kg IV push or IC.
- Calcium chloride 20 mg/kg slow IV push or IC.
- Lidocaine 0.5–1 mg/kg IV push to a maximum of 50 mg per dose every 20 minutes.

Digoxin should not be given to children.

When defibrillating a child, use pediatric paddles or the anterior posterior paddle placement; administer 3.5–6.0 w/s per kg of body weight, up to 50 kg; over 50 kg use full output of the defibrillator.

Transport

- Monitor closely enroute.
- Watch drip rate on IV drugs; watch for side effects.
- No need for Code 3 if patient is stabilized.

ASTHMA

History

- When did the respiratory difficulty start?
- Is the patient having trouble with inspiration? Expiration?
- Did it come on suddenly?
- What provoked the attack?
- Has this happened before?

- Has the patient taken any medications? When?
- What usually breaks the attack?

Physical Exam

- What is the respiratory status?
- What is the level of consciousness?
- What is the skin color, temperature, and moisture?
- What are the patient's vital signs?
- Are wheezes or rales audible on auscultation?
- Are there any physical findings that might indicate allergic reaction or congestive heart failure?
- What is the EKG pattern?

Differential Diagnosis

Rule out allergic reaction and upper airway obstruction. Can be confused with:

- Congestive heart failure, pulmonary edema (cardiac asthma)
- Bronchitis, emphysema
- Spontaneous pneumothorax
- Pulmonary embolus
- Hyperventilation syndrome

Treatment

1. Ensure airway and give humidified oxygen, high-flow.
2. Allow patient to assume position of comfort (usually upright).
3. Give Isuprel inhalant (if not already taken by patient).
4. Give Epinephrine 1:1,000 0.3 mg SC; may repeat.
5. Start an IV of D$_5$W TKO.
6. Give Aminophylline 250–500 mg in 20 ml (IV Volutrol) over 20–30 minutes if Epinephrine is not effective.

7. May hydrate the patient with IV or oral fluids.

Special Note

- It is often helpful to move the patient into the ambulance and out of the public eye before treating; a quiet environment helps to calm the patient.
- If the patient took medication prior to arrival of the paramedics, bring in the container.

Pediatric Note

- Pediatric dosage of Epinephrine 1:1,000 is 0.1 mg SC, up to 0.3 mg
- Aminophylline should be used with caution in children under 12 years of age.

Transport

- Transport the patient in an upright position and give oxygen.
- If unable to relieve attack, transport the patient immediately.

BEHAVIORAL EMERGENCIES

History

- Exactly what happened?
- What was the patient doing at the time?
- When did this occur and how long did it persist?
- Has this happened before?
- What behavior is the patient exhibiting now?
- What is the mental status, including general appearance, affect, thought processes, and cognitive knowledge?
- Is there any indication of trauma?

- Has the patient taken any drugs or been drinking?
- Does the patient take any medications?
- Is there any history of mental illness?
- Is the patient seeing a personal physician?
- Is there any history of diabetes, hypertension, or seizure disorder?

Physical Exam

- Is there any respiratory distress?
- Is the patient hypoxic?
- Is there any sign of head injury or other trauma?
- What is the level of consciousness?
- Is the patient oriented to time, place and person?
- What are the vital signs?
- Is there any pulmonary congestion?
- Are the pupils normal?
- What is the EKG pattern?
- Are there any needle marks?
- Is there a Medic-Alert tag or wallet card?

Differential Diagnosis

Rule out: hypoxia
head injury
drugs
alcohol ingestion
hypoglycemia
CVA

Treatment

1. Ensure ABCs.
2. Use a calm, firm approach with the patient.
3. Give oxygen if hypoxia is suspected.
4. Give 50% dextrose 25 gm IV push if hypoglycemia is suspected.

5. Consider Valium 2.5–20 mg IV push for acute stress reaction.

Special Note

- Patient is often a threat to himself or others. Approach will have to vary with each patient; it may not be practical to attempt history, physical, or extensive treatment on these patients.
- The majority of patient management will come from individual interactions at the scene. It is very likely that communications will be interspersed with long pauses.
- Bring in any samples of ingested drugs, plants, or other causative agents.
- IM medications are of little value in these patients.

Transport

- Restrain only if necessary to prevent injury.
- Avoid unnecessary Code 3 responses, as they usually upset the patient.
- Consider law enforcement assistance if needed.

BURNS

History

- What was the causative agent (heat, chemical, electricity, tar)?
- Where, when, and how did the burn occur?
- Was the patient burned in an enclosed space such as a car or garage?
- What is the patient's age and weight?
- What is the patient's medical history?
- Was any treatment instituted prior to arrival of paramedics?

Physical Exam

- Are there any signs of respiratory distress?
- Are there signs of laryngeal edema?
- Is there any sign suggestive of respiratory involvement such as singed nasal hairs, burns of the face, or soot or blisters in the oropharynx?
- What is the patient's level of consciousness?
- What are the vital signs?
- What are the lung sounds?
- Where are the burns located?
- What is the estimated percentage and degree of the burn injury?
- Are there any associated injuries?
- If *electrical,* is there an entrance or exit wound?
- If *chemical,* what agent was involved?

Differential Diagnosis

- Rule out respiratory involvement
- Rule out carbon monoxide poisoning
- Determine severity of burn:
  Major: over 20% second or third degree
  respiratory involvement
  underlying disease (heart, respiratory)
  Minor: less than 20% second or third degree
  no respiratory involvement
  no complicating factors

Treatment

1. Move patient to a safe environment.
2. Break contact with causative agent (extinguish flames, wash off chemicals).
3. Attend to ABCs; patient may need to be ventilated or may need CPR.
4. Treat any life–threatening injuries.
5. If burn is *Major:*
   - give oxygen, high-flow
   - start an IV of RL, NS, or volume

expanders using a large bore cannula
needle and run to maintain blood
pressure

- give small doses of analgesics if needed
(morphine sulfate in 2 mg increments
IV push, up to 15 mg)

- cover wounds, keep patient warm, and
treat as a shock patient

6. If burn is *Minor:*

- apply cool saline soaks or cold pack to
help alleviate pain

- keep wound clean and covered

- an IV of RL or NS may be started as
a precaution

7. Do not break blisters, remove stuck
clothing, soak wounded area in ice water,
apply any type of ointment, or give any
IM medications.

8. Remove all constricting items such as
rings, necklaces, and bracelets.

For Chemical: Flush immediately with copious amounts of water.
EXCEPTION: If the chemical is dry, brush it off; do not apply
water.

For Electrical: Treat symptomatically. Support cardiovascular
system and monitor closely.

For Respiratory: See Smoke/Gas Inhalation Protocol.

For Tar: Cool with water and transport. Do not attempt to
remove the tar.

Special Note

- Burns do not cause a patient to lose consciousness. If the
patient is unconscious, look for other causes such as head
injury or carbon monoxide poisoning.

Pediatric Note

- Body surface area is estimated differently in children than
adults.

- Burns are one of the more common forms of child abuse.

Transport

- Transport immediately to nearest basic emergency facility if the patient has respiratory involvement.
- Follow triage guidelines to determine most appropriate facility for care.
- Any burn of a critical area such as hands, feet, face, or perineum should be transported for medical evaluation regardless of how small the affected area.

CARDIAC ARREST

History

- What happened?
- How long has the patient been down?
- What is the patient's age and weight?
- Does the patient have any terminal illness?
- Does the patient have a history of heart problems or other medical illnesses?
- Is the patient on any medications?
- What was the patient doing at the time of the attack?
- Was any treatment instituted prior to the arrival of the paramedics?

Physical Exam

- What is the patient's level of consciousness (shake and shout)?
- Is the patient breathing?
- What is the carotid pulse?
- What is the skin color, temperature, and moisture?
- What rhythm does the EKG paddle–check show?
- Are there any obvious injuries?

Differential Diagnosis

- Evaluate respirations and major pulses to determine if the patient is unconscious or has actually arrested.

Treatment

1. Open airway and begin mouth-to-mouth resuscitation.
2. Ventilate with 100% oxygen.
3. If monitored (witnessed) arrest, administer precordial thump within one minute of arrest.
4. Begin cardiac compressions.
5. Control major bleeding.
6. Insert an esophageal obturator airway or endotracheal tube.
7. Start an IV of D_5W TKO.
8. Administer 1 mEq/kg of sodium bicarbonate initially; this dose can be repeated. Thereafter one-half the initial dose can be given at 10 minute intervals.
9. Treat arrhythmias according to separate protocol.
10. Treat underlying cause of arrest.
11. To support cardiovascular system, give:
    - Dopamine 400–800 mg in 250–500 ml D_5W, *or*
    - Aramine 0.5 mg *slow* IV push or 100–200 mg in 250–500 ml D_5W, *or*
    - Levophed 4–8 mg in 250–500 ml D_5W, titrate to blood pressure and patient condition.

Special Note

- Cardiac arrest following trauma is usually accompanied by hypovolemia and should be concurrently treated with antishock procedures.
- Assess pupils and peripheral pulses during resuscitation.

Pediatric Note

- Pediatric doses:
  Sodium bicarbonate 1mEq/kg IV push
  Dopamine 200 mg in 500 ml of D_5W; begin with

5 μgm/kg/min; titrate to blood pressure

Aramine 0.01 mg/kg IV push, *or* 50–100 mg in 250–500 ml D₅W, titrate to blood pressure

Levophed 2–4 mg in 250–500 ml D₅W IV drip, titrate to blood pressure

- Children remain viable longer than adults, so may institute CPR even if the child has been down longer than 4–6 minutes.
- Precordial thump is not recommended on children.

Transport

- Transport Code 3 as soon as possible.

CEREBROVASCULAR ACCIDENT

History

- When did the problem start?
- What was the patient doing when the symptoms occurred?
- Did the patient have any headache, dizziness, or chest pain prior to the episode?
- Does the patient have any predisposing factors such as hypertension, atherosclerosis, prior CVAs or TIAs, recent illnesses or surgeries?
- Has the patient been taking any medication?
- Did the patient lose consciousness; if so, for how long?
- Has there been any change in level of consciousness since the symptoms began?
- Did the patient fall and possibly injure himself?
- Does the patient have a history of atrial fibrillation?

Physical Exam

- What is the respiratory status?
- What is the patient's level of consciousness?

- What is the patient's neurological status (pupils, hand grasps, movement of extremities)?
- Is there any facial paralysis or difficulty speaking or swallowing?
- Has the patient been incontinent of urine or stool?
- What are the vital signs, lung sounds, skin color, temperature, and moisture?
- What is the EKG pattern?
- Is there any evidence of trauma?

Differential Diagnosis

- If the patient is unconscious, rule out other causes of coma.

Treatment

1. Ensure airway and give oxygen.
2. If patient is having difficulty with secretions, position on affected side and suction secretions.
3. Start an IV of D_5W TKO.
4. Reassure patient, especially if experiencing aphasia.

Transport

- Protect airway and watch for change in patient status.

CHEST PAIN
(Nontraumatic)

History

- When did the chest pain start?
- How does the patient describe the pain?
- How severe is the pain?

- Where is the pain located, and does it radiate to arms, back, neck, or jaw?
- What was the patient doing when the pain started?
- Is the pain associated with respiration or difficulty breathing?
- Does anything make the pain better or worse?
- Has this ever happened before?
- What is the patient's medical history?
- Is the patient on any medication?
- Has the patient taken anything for the pain?
- Is the patient nauseated?

Physical Exam

- Is the patient breathing effectively?
- What is the patient's level of consciousness?
- What is the skin color, moisture, and temperature?
- What are the vital signs?
- What is the EKG pattern?
- What are the lung sounds?
- Are there any signs of CHF such as distended neck veins or peripheral edema?

Differential Diagnosis

Rule out trauma
Consider the following:
- Myocardial infarction
- Pulmonary embolus
- Pleurisy
- Aneurysm
- Pericarditis
- Pneumonia
- Spontaneous pneumothorax
- Hyperventilation

Treatment

For suspected *angina pectoris:*
1. Give high-flow oxygen.
2. If not hypotensive, may administer nitroglycerin 0.4 mg (1/150 gr) sublingually.
3. If no relief from nitroglycerin, give morphine sulfate 2–15 mg IV push in 2 mg increments until desired effect.

For a suspected *myocardial infarction:*
1. Give high-flow oxygen if not contra-indicated.
2. Start an IV of D₅W TKO.
3. Treat arrhythmias according to separate protocol.
4. Give morphine sulfate 2–15 mg in 2 mg increments IV push, titrate to relief of pain.
5. Give lidocaine 50–100 mg IV push prophylactically; follow with IV drip of 1–2 gm in 250/500 ml D₅W, adjust flow rate to 1–2 mg/min.
6. If patient is in cardiogenic shock, administer:
   - Dopamine 400–800 mg in 250–500 ml D₅W, *or*
   - Aramine 0.5 mg *slow* IV push or 100–200 mg in 250–500 ml D₅W, *or*
   - Levophed 4–8 mg in 250–500 ml D₅W titrate to blood pressure and patient condition.
7. Reassure patient.

For a suspected *aneurysm:*
1. Give high-flow oxygen.
2. Start an IV of RL or NS using a large bore cannula needle and run to maintain blood pressure.
3. Transport Code 3 without delay.

4. Consider application of antishock trousers.

For a suspected *respiratory disorder:*
See specific protocol.

Special Note

- Patients who complain of chest pain in the field should be suspected of having an MI and be treated accordingly unless evidence negates this possibility.
- Cardiogenic shock carries a high mortality rate and warrants immediate attention.

Transport

- Do not use Code 3 unless condition is critical.
- Allow patient to assume position of comfort.

CHEST TRAUMA

History

- What was the mechanism of injury?
- What is the nature and extent of the injuries?
- Is the patient having any respiratory distress?
- Is he having trouble getting air in or out?
- Is there any pain; if so, where?
- Is the pain associated with breathing?
- Is there any cough or hemoptysis?
- Is there any active bleeding; if so, what is the estimated blood loss?
- Does the patient have any major medical illnesses?

Physical Exam

- Is the airway adequate?
- Are the respirations effective?

- Are there any open chest wounds?
- Is major bleeding controlled?
- Is there any paradoxical respiration, intercostal indrawing, tracheal deviation, or neck vein distention?
- What is the patient's level of consciousness?
- What is the skin color, moisture, and temperature?
- What are the vital signs?
- What are the lung sounds?
- What is the EKG pattern?
- What are the associated injuries?

Differential Diagnosis

Consider:
Open chest wounds
Flail chest
Pneumothorax
Hemothorax
Cardiac tamponade
Tension pneumothorax
Fractured ribs
Crushed trachea
Bleeding from major intrathoracic vessels
Myocardial trauma

Treatment

1. Open airway, ventilate if necessary.
2. Give high-flow oxygen.
3. Control active bleeding.
4. Start an IV of RL, NS, or volume expanders using a large bore cannula needle, run to maintain blood pressure.
5. Position patient to facilitate respiratory exchange.
6. Do not administer analgesics.
7. Stabilize spine and splint fractures.

Open chest wound: Cover with Vaseline gauze but watch for the development of tension pneumothorax; remove dressing briefly if this occurs, then reapply and observe closely.

Flail chest: Stabilize chest wall with sandbags and ventilate with positive pressure respirator.

Pneumothorax/hemothorax: Ventilate with high-flow oxygen and transport as soon as possible.

Tension pneumothorax: Perform a needle thoracostomy or transport immediately Code 3.

Cardiac tamponade: Perform a pericardiocentesis or transport immediately Code 3.

Special Note

- Do not delay at the scene; expedite the run and transport as quickly as possible since these patients are highly unstable.

Transport

- Monitor patient very closely enroute, especially respiratory status.

CHRONIC OBSTRUCTIVE PULMONARY DISEASE (COPD)

History

- When did the problem start?
- Has the patient ever had this problem before?
- Does the patient have a history of lung disease?
- What brought on the attack?
- Is the patient having trouble getting air in or out?
- What was the patient doing when the attack came on?
- Has the patient had any recent respiratory infection?
- Is the patient on any medications?
- Did the patient take any medications today?
- What usually breaks the attack?
- Is the patient having any pain?
- Is the pain related to respiration?
- Does the patient have a cough?
- Is the cough productive; if so, what is it like?

Physical Exam

- What is the effectiveness of respirations?
- Are the respirations noisy?
- What is the level of consciousness?
- What is the skin color, moisture, and temperature?
- What are the vital signs?
- What lung sounds are heard on auscultation?
- What is the EKG rhythm?
- Is the patient using any accessory muscles to breathe?
- Are the neck veins distended?
- Does the patient have a barrel chest?
- Is there any peripheral edema?

Differential Diagnosis

- Must differentiate an acute attack of chronic lung disease from CHF and other respiratory emergencies.
- Do not overlook the possibility of an MI.

Treatment

1. Assure airway and ventilate if necessary.
2. Give low-flow oxygen at 2–3 liters/min.
3. Place patient in upright position or position of comfort.
4. Start an IV of D₅W TKO.
5. May give Isuprel inhalant or Amino-phylline 250–500 mg IV Volutrol in 20 ml of solution over 20–30 minutes depending upon severity of respiratory distress.

Special Note

- Administer low-flow oxygen to all COPD patients.
- If patient condition is deteriorating despite 2–3 liters of oxygen, may increase concentration gradually, but be prepared to assist ventilations.

Transport

- Keep patient in position of comfort, usually upright or leaning forward with arms on pillow.
- Use Code 3 only if patient condition indicates it.

COLD INJURIES

History

- What is the mechanism of injury (chemical, wet, dry, refrigeration, environmental)?
- What was the length of exposure to the cold?
- What precipitated the injury (fall, overdose, unconsciousness)?
- Was any treatment begun prior to the arrival of the paramedics?

Physical Exam

- Are the patient's respirations and circulation adequate?
- What is the patient's level of consciousness?
- What is the appearance of the exposed area (mottled, swollen, reddened, pale, blistered, necrotic)?
- Is there any feeling or movement of the area?
- What are the patient's vital signs?
- What does the EKG show?

Differential Diagnosis

- Rule out underlying contributing factors such as alcohol, overdose, cardiac condition.

Treatment

1. Administer oxygen and assist ventilations if necessary.
2. Remove wet clothing.
3. Institute gentle warming with blankets or warm packs; do not apply heat directly to the skin or rub the injured area.

4. Apply dressings to blistered or necrotic areas.
5. If severe, may require cardiovascular support (IV, CPR, drug therapy).

Special Note

- If the patient arrests from profound hypothermia, the time of biological death may be extended up to 10 minutes due to the slower metabolic rate.
- Once re-warming has begun, do not allow injured areas to become cold again.

Transport

- If patient is stable, no need for Code 3 transport.

COMA

History

- How long has the patient been unconscious?
- What occurred immediately before the patient lost consciousness?
- Is there any evidence of trauma?
- Is there any evidence of drug/alcohol ingestion?
- Is there evidence of gas inhalation?
- Is there a Medic–Alert tag or wallet card, or any other medical history?
- Are there any environmental clues such as bottles or syringes?

Physical Exam

- What is the respiratory rate, rhythm, and effectiveness?
- Are there any peripheral pulses?
- What is the level of consciousness?
- What is the skin color, moisture, and temperature?
- What are the vital signs?
- What does the EKG show?
- What does the lung auscultation reveal?

- What are the pupils like?
- Is there an odor to the patient's breath?
- Are there any signs of trauma, needle tracks, or bites?
- Was the patient incontinent of urine or stool?

Differential Diagnosis

Common causes of coma include:
- Diabetic imbalances
- Drug/alcohol overdose
- Trauma
- Neurological disorder such as CVA or seizure

Other causes of coma include:
- Cardiac arrhythmias
- Poisoning
- Behavioral problems

Treatment

1. Assure airway while keeping spine immobilized and suction as needed.
2. Give high-flow oxygen and ventilate if necessary.
3. Control active bleeding.
4. Perform CPR as needed.
5. Perform venipuncture for blood sugar analysis.
6. Start an IV of D$_5$W TKO; if hypovolemia is suspected, start RL or NS and run to maintain blood pressure.
7. Give Narcan 0.4 mg IV push, IM or sublingual; may repeat as many as 10 times to elicit response.
8. Administer 25 gm 50% Dextrose IV push; may repeat.
9. Treat any associated injuries.
10. If patient doesn't respond, immobilize the spine, give supportive care, and transport immediately.

Special Note

- Field treatment is directed at differentiating between hypoglycemia and narcotic overdose, because these are the two major causes of coma which have specific field treatment. If the patient doesn't respond to these diagnostic/treatment measures, transport immediately for further evaluation.

Pediatric Note

- Coma in a child should suggest poisoning, diabetes, child abuse, or neurological disorders.
- Pediatric dosages:
  Narcan 0.005 mg/kg IV push, IM, or sublingual, may repeat as necessary.
  25% Dextrose 0.5–1 gm/kg slow IV push.

Transport

- No need for Code 3 if patient is stabilized.

DIABETES

History

- What are the symptoms?
- When did the symptoms begin?
- Is the patient on oral hypoglycemic agents or other drugs; if so, what kind?
- When did the patient last take medication?
- When did the patient last eat?
- Did the patient lose consciousness, fall, or injure himself?
- Was there any seizure activity?
- Is there any other medical history?

Physical Exam

- Is the airway intact?
- Are the respirations effective?
- What is the level of consciousness?

- What is the skin color, moisture, and temperature?
- What are the vital signs?
- What are the pupils like?
- What does the EKG show?
- Is there an odor to the breath?

Differential Diagnosis

Might be confused with
- head trauma
- alcohol or drug ingestion
- ASA overdose
- hypovolemia
- arrhythmias
- seizure disorder
- behavioral disorder

Treatment

1. Ensure airway and ventilate as needed.
2. Give oxygen.
3. Perform venipuncture for blood sugar analysis.
4. If patient is alert and has a gag reflex, give Glucola 210 ml (75 gm) orally.
5. If patient is unconscious or has no gag reflex, start an IV of D5W TKO and give 50% Dextrose 25 gm IV push; may repeat if necessary.
6. If unable to start an IV, may give Instant Glucose Paste, 12.5 gm (½ tube) between teeth and cheek; may repeat if necessary.
7. Treat any associated injuries.

Special Note

- It is not necessary to differentiate between hypoglycemia and hyperglycemia, because no distinction is made in the field treatment.
- When using Instant Glucose Paste, watch for possible aspiration.

Pediatric Note

Pediatric dose
- 25% Dextrose 0.5-1 g/kg slow IV push
- Glucola 30–210 ml, varies with weight
- Instant Glucose Paste, 12.5 g orally

Transport

- Sometimes these patients are treated in the field and do not want to go to the hospital. Convince them of the need for followup care.

DROWNING

History

- How long was the patient in the water?
- Was he pulled from the surface or the bottom of the water?
- What was his condition when he was pulled from the water?
- How old is the patient?
- Are there any underlying medical problems?
- Are there any drugs or alcohol on board?
- What type of water was involved (salt, fresh, clean, hot, cold, chlorinated)?
- What care was administered prior to the arrival of the paramedics?

Physical Exam

- What is the respiratory status?
- What is the cardiovascular status?
- What is the level of consciousness?
- What are the vital signs?
- What does the EKG show?
- Are there any abnormal lung sounds?

- Are there any associated injuries (especially spinal cord)?
- Did the patient vomit?

Differential Diagnosis

- Was there any underlying cause for the accident such as an MI, hypoglycemia, anaphylaxis, seizure, or trauma?

Treatment

1. Assure airway while keeping spine immobilized and assist ventilations with positive pressure ventilator.
2. Give high-concentration oxygen.
3. Control any severe bleeding.
4. Suction vomitus as needed.
5. Start an IV of D_5W TKO.
6. Treat arrhythmias according to separate protocols.
7. If symptomatic, give sodium bicarbonate 1mEq/kg IV push initially; this dose can be repeated. Thereafter, one-half the initial dose can be given at 10 minute intervals.
8. Keep patient warm.
9. Insert an NG tube to decompress the stomach.
10. Immobilize the spine and splint fractures as indicated.
11. Treat any associated injuries.

Special Note

- Bring a sample of the water to the hospital if possible.
- All near-drowning patients should receive high-flow oxygen and be transported due to the possibility of delayed complications.
- Do not attempt to evacuate water from the lungs.

Pediatric Note

- Pediatric dosage for sodium bicarbonate is 1 mEq/kg IV push.
- Pediatric patients are more resilient than adults, so do not discontinue resuscitation prematurely.

Transport

- Use Code 3 for an unstable patient and continue treatment enroute.

HEAT EXPOSURE

History

- What environment is the patient in (temperature, humidity)?
- How long has the patient been in this environment?
- Does the patient have any pain?
- Does the patient have any vomiting or muscle cramps?
- Did the patient lose consciousness; if so, for how long?
- Did the patient have any seizures?
- Does the patient have any medical problems?
- Is the patient on any medications?

Physical Exam

- Is the patient in respiratory distress?
- What is the patient's level of consciousness?
- What is the skin color, temperature, and moisture?
- What are the vital signs?
- Does the patient have signs of dehydration or shock?
- What is the EKG pattern?

Differential Diagnosis

- Heat cramps
- Heat exhaustion

- Heat stroke
- Sunburn
- Anaphylaxis
- Hypoglycemia

Treatment

1. Assure that airway is open.
2. Administer high-flow oxygen and assist ventilations as necessary.
3. Move patient into the shade.
4. Remove excess clothing.
5. *For heat exhaustion,* cool patient gradually with lukewarm water; prevent shivering.
6. *For heat stroke,* institute rapid cooling measures
   a. ice packs to major artery sites
   b. sponge patient with cold water.
7. Start an IV of RL or NS to replace lost volume.
8. Assess vital signs.
9. Do not give patient any fluids orally.
10. If suspect heat stroke, be prepared for seizures. May administer Valium 2.5–20 mg IV push in 2.5 mg increments.

Special Note

- Heat stroke is a true field emergency and requires immediate intervention.

Pediatric Note

- Check fontanels for dehydration.
- Pediatric dose of Valium is 0.05 mg/kg IV push up to 10 mg.

Transport

- Continue cooling measures enroute.

HYPERVENTILATION SYNDROME

History

- When did the problem start?
- What was the patient doing at the time of onset?
- Has it ever happened before?
- Is the patient having trouble getting air in or out?
- Is the patient having any pain?
- Is the patient light–headed or having any tingling in fingertips or around the mouth?
- Does the patient have any history of cardiac or respiratory problems?
- Has the patient had any recent exposure to toxins, allergens, or foreign substances?
- Is the patient on any medications?
- Is the patient under any emotional stress?

Physical Exam

- How effective are respirations?
- Are there any abnormal respiratory sounds?
- What is the level of consciousness?
- What is the skin color, moisture, and temperature?
- What are the vital signs?
- What lung sounds are heard on auscultation?
- What is the EKG pattern?

Differential Diagnosis

- Rule out trauma, overdose (especially ASA), or diabetic ketoacidosis.
- Can be confused with many other cardiopulmonary disorders.
- Be sure to eliminate organic causes before labeling it an emotional reaction.

Treatment

1. Reassure and calm patient.
2. Have patient breathe slowly into a paper bag.

Special Note

- When in doubt, assume the patient has an organic problem and give treatment accordingly.

Transport

- If patient does not respond to treatment, should be evaluated at the hospital to rule out a medical disorder.

MARINE INJURIES

History

- What kind of marine animal was the patient in contact with?
- Is there any pain; if so, what is it like?
- When did the injury occur?
- When did the patient begin having symptoms?
- Does the patient have a history of allergies?
- Is there a history of cardiac problems?
- Does the patient have any abdominal cramps, vomiting, or tingling?

Physical Exam

- Is there any difficulty breathing?
- What is the level of consciousness?
- What are the lung sounds like?
- What is the skin color, moisture, temperature?
- Are there any lacerations, sting marks, welts, or hives?
- Is there any swelling?

- What are the vital signs?
- What is the EKG pattern?

Differential Diagnosis

- Identify the causative agent (stingray, jellyfish).
- Distinguish between local and systemic reaction.

Treatment

1. Ensure airway.
2. If injury is *jellyfish sting,* rinse with alcohol; a cool compress may alleviate pain.
3. If *stingray injury,* remove barb if possible; apply heat locally.
4. If systemic response begins:
   a. apply constricting band proximal to the site
   b. give oxygen
   c. give Epinephrine 1:1000, 0.3 mg SC may repeat; may also give 0.1 mg at site if other than fingers or toes
   d. start an IV of D₅W TKO
5. Reassure patient; keep him calm.

Special Note

- If severe reaction is occurring, consider intubation.
- Do not give analgesics for pain.

Pediatric Note

- Pediatric dose of Epinephrine 1:1000 is 0.1 mg s.c. up to 0.3 mg.

Transport

- No need for Code 3 transportation if patient is stabilized.

NEUROLOGICAL TRAUMA

History

- When did the accident occur?
- What was the mechanism of injury?
- Was the patient ever unconscious; if so, was it immediate with the injury or was there a lucid interval?
- What was the patient doing prior to the accident?
- Is there any evidence of alcohol or drugs on board?
- Are there any associated injuries?

Physical Exam

- Are respirations compromised in any way?
- Is there any obvious bleeding?
- What is the level of consciousness?
- Is the patient oriented to time, place, and person?
- Are there any signs of shock (pulse, blood pressure, skin color, moisture, and temperature)?
- What are the pupils like?
- Is there any fluid or blood in the ears or nose?
- Is the patient able to move all extremities?
- Does the patient have any head, neck, back, or shoulder pain?
- What are the findings of a head-to-toe exam?
- Is there any decorticate or decerebrate posturing?

Differential Diagnosis

Consider other conditions which may mimic neurological trauma:
- Alcohol or drug ingestion
- Postictal state
- Diabetes
- Cerebrovascular accident

Treatment

1. Assure an airway while keeping spine immobilized; assist ventilations if necessary.
2. Give high-flow oxygen.
3. Suction airway as needed.
4. Control any severe bleeding.
5. Start an IV of RL or NS and run it at a TKO rate; if hypovolemia is present, run IV to maintain blood pressure.
6. If signs of increased intracranial pressure occur, consider the use of diuretics or steroids.
7. If low-resistance shock is present, may give
   a. Levophed 4–8 mg in 250–500 ml of D$_5$W, or
   b. Aramine 0.5 mg slow IV push, or 100–200 mg in 250–500 ml of D$_5$W, or
   c. Dopamine 400–800 mg in 250–500 ml D$_5$W, titrate to maintain blood pressure.
8. In low-resistance shock that does not respond to drug therapy, antishock trousers may be applied.
9. Do not give analgesics.
10. Stabilize head and spine.

Special Note

- All head injuries should be suspected of having associated spinal cord injury; all such cases should be immobilized before moving.
- Neurological trauma can cause low–resistance shock and require cardiovascular support.
- Unless hypovolemia is present, run IV at a TKO rate to avoid increasing intracranial pressure.

Pediatric Note

- Check for bulging fontanels.
- Pediatric Doses:

- Aramine 0.01 mg/kg IV push, or 50–100 mg in 250 ml of D₅W, titrate to blood pressure.
- Dopamine 200 mg in 500 ml D₅W; begin drip at 5 μgm/kg/min.
- Mannitol 250 mg/kg/IV drip per Volutrol over 5 min.
- Levophed 4 mg/500 ml D₅W; titrate to BP.

Transport

- Do *not* delay in the field.
- If patient condition is deteriorating, transport immediately Code 3 and institute treatment enroute.

OBSTETRICAL EMERGENCIES

History

- Which pregnancy is this?
- What is the due date?
- Has the mother had any trouble with previous pregnancies/deliveries?
- Has the mother had any trouble with this pregnancy?
- Have the membranes ruptured?
- Is the amniotic fluid meconium–stained?
- When did the contractions start?
- What is the frequency, regularity, and duration of the contractions?
- Has the patient had prenatal care; by whom?
- Does the patient have any medical problems?
- Is the patient on any medications?
- Does the patient have any pain other than the contractions?

Physical Exam

- Are the mother's respirations adequate?
- Is the baby crowning with contractions?
- Are any presenting parts visible in the birth canal; if so, which parts are presenting first?

- Is there any bloody show or frank bleeding?
- What is the mother's skin color, temperature, and moisture?
- What are the vital signs?
- Does the mother have any peripheral edema?

Differential Diagnosis

- Determine if delivery is imminent or if there is time to transport.
- Consider possible complications such as eclampsia, placenta previa, abruptio placenta, twins, breech delivery, or prolapsed cord.

Treatment

If there is no time for transport, the paramedic will proceed with the delivery:

1. Ensure the mother's ABCs.
2. Administer oxygen.
3. Start an IV of RL or NS if time allows; run at a TKO rate.
4. Suction the baby's airway as soon as the head is delivered.
5. Allow delivery to continue normally.
6. Assess baby for Apgar score.
7. If baby is in distress, resuscitate as needed.
8. Put the baby to the mother's breast and keep warm.
9. Allow placenta to deliver; do not pull on cord.
10. Once placenta is delivered, bleeding can be controlled by massaging the fundus.
11. Administer Pitocin 3–10 units IM or 10–20 units in 1000 cc RL or NS titrated to control uterine bleeding.
12. If mother is bleeding heavily and exhibiting signs of shock, massage fundus, increase IV flow rate, place in shock position, and transport.

Special Note

- If birth is breech, allow infant to deliver to the waist without active assistance (give support only); once the legs and buttocks are delivered, the head can be assisted out. If head does not deliver within 4–6 minutes, insert a gloved hand into the vagina and create an airway for the infant.

- If the cord is wrapped around the infant's neck, slip the cord over the head and off the neck; may need to clamp and cut the cord if it is tightly wrapped.

- In case of prolapsed cord, place the mother in a shock position with her hips elevated on pillows, insert a gloved hand into the vagina and gently push the baby's head off the cord. *Transport Code 3 while retaining this position; do not remove hand until relieved by hospital personnel.*

- If the mother is eclamptic and having seizures, consider Valium 2.5–20 mg slow IV push in 2.5 mg increments over 1 minute. Use Valium cautiously as it may cause respiratory depression in the baby as well as the mother. Transport quickly, but keep environment dark and quiet; do NOT use Code 3.

- Two common causes of bleeding during pregnancy are abruptio placenta and placenta previa. For either of these conditions, start an IV of RL or NS and run it to maintain blood pressure. Place patient in shock position, keep her warm, and transport immediately. Do *not* use Pitocin.

- Consider the possibility of pregnancy in any female who is of reproductive age and complains of vaginal bleeding or abdominal pain.

- Multiple births are an unusual but possible occurrence. Be aware of that possibility and stay with the mother following the first delivery.

Transport

- With any birth that is difficult or not progressing, transport if at all possible.

- Keep the baby warm at all times; monitor respirations closely.

- Reassess baby and mother frequently.

OVERDOSE

History

- What did the patient take?
- Did the patient mix any substances?
- How much did the patient take?
- When was the agent injected/ingested?
- When did the symptoms start?
- If unconscious, how long has he been unconscious?
- Has this occurred before?
- Did the patient vomit?
- Did the patient have a seizure?
- Has the patient been drinking?
- Has the patient had any medical problems?
- Is the patient on any prescribed medication?

Physical Exam

- What is the respiratory status?
- Is there obvious trauma or bleeding?
- What is the level of consciousness?
- What is the skin temperature, color, and moisture?
- What are the vital signs?
- What are the pupils like?
- What does the EKG monitor show?
- What are the lung sounds?
- Are there any track marks?
- Is there any odor to the breath?

Differential Diagnosis

Rule out:
- Diabetes
- Cardiovascular problem
- Anaphylaxis
- Trauma
- Asphyxiation

Treatment

1. Assure the airway, ventilate as needed, and administer high-flow oxygen.
2. If patient is alert and has a gag reflex, give Syrup of Ipecac 30 ml orally, followed by several large glasses of water.
3. Establish an IV of D5W TKO.
4. If patient is unconscious or has respiratory depression, administer Narcan 0.4 mg IV push IM or sublingual, may repeat as many as 10 times to elicit response.
5. If patient has been apneic, administer sodium bicarbonate 1 mEq/kg IV push.
6. Suction as needed.

Special Note

- Do not insert an esophageal airway if Narcan is to be used.
- If patient vomits, bring sample to the hospital.
- Bring in all empty containers and syringes.

Pediatric Note

Pediatric dosages:
- Syrup of Ipecac: 15 ml orally
- Narcan: 0.005 mg/kg IV push or IM
- 25% Dextrose: 0.5-1 g/kg slow IV push
- Sodium bicarbonate: 1 mEq/kg IV push

Transport

- Transport Code 3 if patient status deteriorates.
- Observe patient closely for respiratory depression and/or decreasing level of consciousness.
- May have to repeat Narcan enroute.

POISONING

History

- What did the patient take or come in contact with?
- Did the patient mix any substances?
- How much was taken?
- When did the patient take it?
- When did the symptoms begin?
- Did the patient vomit?
- What was the vomitus like?
- Is there any headache, dizziness, hallucination or visual disturbance?

Physical Exam

- What is the respiratory status?
- Is there any laryngeal edema, stridor, cyanosis, cough, or pulmonary congestion?
- Are there any blisters on the lips or in the mouth or oropharynx?
- What is the patient's level of consciousness?
- What is the skin moisture, temperature, and color?
- What are the vital signs?
- Is there any parasympathetic effect such as increased salivation, tearing, urination, or bradycardia?
- Is there any muscle tremor, or seizure activity?
- Is there any nausea, vomiting, or abdominal cramping?
- What is the EKG pattern?

Differential Diagnosis

- Consider hypoglycemia or neurological disorder.
- Distinguish between caustic and noncaustic ingestions.

Treatment

1. Ensure airway and assist ventilations if needed.
2. Suction as needed.
3. Give high-flow oxygen if symptoms are significant.
4. If substance was exposed to the skin, remove clothing and rinse patient with copious amounts of water.
5. If the patient is alert and has a gag reflex, and the substance is known to be noncaustic, give Syrup of Ipecac 30 ml orally with large amounts of water.
6. Start an IV of D₅W TKO.
7. If *organophosphate poisoning,* give Atropine 2 mg IV push or IM; may repeat every 3–8 minutes as needed.
8. If overdose of *tricyclic antidepressants,* and patient is psychotic, hallucinating, and/or having cardiac arrhythmias, give Physostigmine 2 mg in 10 ml IV Volutrol over 2 minutes; may repeat at 5-minute intervals.
9. If *caustic* agent, do *not* induce vomiting. Give milk, provide supportive measures, and transport.

Special Note

- Save any empty containers or samples and bring to hospital.
- Rescuers should protect themselves from contact with topical powders.
- If patient vomits, bring sample to the hospital.
- Watch patient's airway if Syrup of Ipecac is used.
- Call Poison Center for specific directions.

Pediatric Note

Pediatric doses:
- Physostigmine: 0.5 mg–2 mg in 10 ml IV Volutrol over 2-minute period.

- Syrup of Ipecac: 15 ml orally.
- Atropine 0.05 mg/kg IV push; may repeat every 3–8 minutes.

Accidental poisoning is extremely common in toddlers.

Transport

- Code 3 should be used if patient ingested a caustic substance or is deteriorating rapidly.

PULMONARY EDEMA

History

- How severe is the dyspnea?
- When did it start?
- What brought on the attack?
- Has this ever happened before?
- Is the patient having trouble getting air in or out?
- Is there any associated chest pain?
- Is there any history of cardiac or respiratory disorders?
- Does the patient have respiratory difficulty at night?
- Is the patient on any medications or special diet; if so, has the patient been adhering to these?

Physical Exam

- Is the patient breathing effectively?
- Does the patient have noisy respirations?
- What is the level of consciousness?
- Does the patient have pink frothy sputum?
- What is the skin color, temperature, and moisture?
- What are the vital signs?
- What are the lung sounds on auscultation?
- What is the EKG pattern?
- Does the patient have distended neck veins or peripheral edema?

Differential Diagnosis

- Rule out MI
- Can be confused with:
    Emphysema
    Bronchitis
    Asthma
    Pulmonary embolus
    Pneumonia
    Anaphylaxis
    Obstructed airway

Treatment

1. Give high-flow oxygen unless the patient has COPD.
2. Place patient in position of comfort.
3. Give positive pressure ventilation if condition is severe.
4. Start an IV of D5W TKO.
5. Give Lasix 20–80 mg IV push.
6. Give morphine sulfate 2–15 mg IV push in 2 mg increments.
7. Give Aminophylline 250–500 mg in 20 ml IV Volutrol over 20–30 minutes.
8. Give Lanoxin 0.25–0.5 mg slow IV push.
9. Apply rotating tourniquets (may apply sooner if unable to start IV).
10. Give reassurance.
11. Treat associated arrhythmias as they arise.

Special Note

- Suctioning is often ineffective.

Transport

- Monitor patient closely.
- Transport in upright position.

RAPE

History

- What happened?
- When did the attack occur?
- Is there obvious trauma?
- Is there any vaginal or rectal bleeding or discharge?
- Does the patient have pain anywhere?
- How old is the patient?
- What did the patient do after the attack?

Physical Exam

- What is the respiratory status?
- What is the level of consciousness and emotional state?
- Are there any signs of hypovolemic shock?
- What are the vital signs?
- Are there any bruises or lacerations?
- Are there any broken bones?

Differential Diagnosis

- Look for associated injuries.
- Consider hypovolemia.

Treatment

1. Assure airway and administer oxygen.
2. Control any obvious bleeding.
3. Start an IV of RL or NS if fluid replacement is needed.
4. Splint any fractures.

Special Note

- Do not allow patient to bathe or change clothes.
- Give emotional support.

Pediatric Note

- Much more likely to have associated trauma.
- Watch closely for hypovolemia.

Transport

- If patient is stable, no need to transport Code 3.

SEIZURES

History

- Is the patient still seizing?
- When did the seizure start?
- What was the seizure like?
- How long did it last?
- Has this ever happened before?
- Does the patient have a diagnosed seizure disorder?
- Is the patient on any medications; has he been taking them regularly; has the prescription been changed recently?
- Did the patient fall and possibly hurt himself?
- Did the patient regain consciousness immediately?
- Is the patient pregnant?
- Has the patient been exposed to any noxious chemicals?

Physical Exam

- What is the respiratory status?
- What is the patient's level of consciousness?
- Are there any lacerations of the tongue, head, or extremities?
- What is skin color, moisture, and temperature?
- What are the vital signs?
- What are the pupils like?
- What does the EKG show?

- Has the patient been incontinent?
- Are there any signs of paralysis, weakness, or unequal grips?
- Does the patient have a Medic–Alert tag or wallet card?

Differential Diagnosis

Although epilepsy is the most common cause of seizures, other possible causes include:

- Hypoxia
- Cardiac arrhythmias
- Hypoglycemia
- Drug/alcohol withdrawal
- Poison/drug ingestion
- Meningitis/encephalitis
- Head injuries

Treatment

1. Ensure airway, give oxygen, and suction as needed.
2. Start an IV of D_5W TKO.
3. Consider $D_{50}W$ 25 gm IV push as a diagnostic measure.
4. Give Valium 2.5–20 mg IV push in 2.5 mg increments to control active, prolonged, or recurrent seizures.
5. Keep patient from injuring himself during seizure.
6. Reassure patient.
7. Treat any resultant injuries.

Special Note

- Watch for respiratory depression if Valium is used.
- A patient in a postictal state may act lethargic, drift off to sleep, or experience short-term memory loss.

Pediatric Note

- In children ages 1–4 years convulsions may occur with high temperature spikes.
- Febrile convulsions should be treated enroute with gentle cooling measures.
- If seizures persist, give Valium 0.05 mg/kg slow IV push; watch for respiratory depression.

Transport

- Watch for recurrence of seizure.
- Protect from injury.

SHOCK
(Hypovolemic)

History

Is there any indication of trauma?
- When did it occur?
- What was the mechanism of injury?
- Does the patient have any pain?
- Where is the pain?
- Has the patient's level of consciousness changed since the incident?
- Is there obvious blood loss; if so, what is the estimated volume?

Does the patient have any current or recent medical problem?
- Has the patient been nauseated or vomited?
- Has the patient vomited blood or coffee–ground material?
- Has the patient had diarrhea or tarry/bloody stools?
- Is the patient febrile?
- Does the patient have any pain; if so, what is it like?
- Does the patient have a past medical history of ulcers, cardiovascular disease, colitis, or hypertension?
- Is the patient on any medications?

Physical Exam

- Does the patient have any respiratory distress?
- Is there any active bleeding?
- What is the level of consciousness?
- What is the skin temperature, moisture, and color?
- What are the vital signs?
- Is there any unusual swelling or hematoma formation?
- Is the abdomen rigid?
- What is the EKG pattern?

Differential Diagnosis

- Rule out cardiogenic shock and low resistance shock.

Treatment

1. Assure airway.
2. Assist ventilations if necessary and administer high-flow oxygen.
3. Control any obvious bleeding.
4. Start an IV of RL or NS and run it to maintain blood pressure.
5. Splint any fractures.
6. Keep the patient warm.
7. Place patient in shock position if not contraindicated.
8. If shock is severe, may require:
   - volume expanders
   - antishock trousers
   - dopamine or vasopressors after fluid replacement

Pediatric Note

- Use a Volutrol to administer IV fluids.
- Check fontanels for dehydration.

Transport

- Transport as soon as possible; monitor EKG and VS enroute.
- If trauma is severe, may transport directly to regional trauma center.
- Watch IVs closely enroute.

SMOKE/GAS INHALATION

History

- What did the patient inhale?
- Where was the patient found?
- Was the patient in an enclosed area?
- How long was the patient exposed?
- Were there any heaters, stoves, ovens, or fires at the scene?
- Was the patient using chemicals to clean?
- Was the patient ever unconscious; if so, what aroused him?
- Does the patient have a headache or other pain?
- Does the patient have any relevant medical history?
- Is the patient on any medications?

Physical Exam

- What is the patient's respiratory status?
- Are the respirations noisy?
- What is the level of consciousness?
- What is the skin color, moisture, and temperature?
- Are there any singed nasal hairs or soot around the face?
- Are there any burns of the patient's face or neck?
- What lung sounds are heard on auscultation?
- What are the vital signs?
- What is the EKG rhythm?
- Are there any neurological findings such as twitching or convulsing?

Differential Diagnosis

- Rule out hypovolemic shock from burns.
- Consider neurological disorder such as subarachnoid hemorrhage or seizure disorder.
- Do not overlook possibility of underlying medical disorder.
- Identify causative agent if at all possible.

Treatment

1. Remove patient from harmful environment (ensure personal safety; wear breathing apparatus if indicated).
2. Ensure patient's airway and assist ventilations if needed.
3. Administer 100% oxygen.
4. Start an IV of D_5W TKO; may use RL or NS if volume replacement is needed.
5. If bronchospasm is present, may give Aminophylline 250–500 mg in 20 ml D_5W IV Volutrol over 20–30 min.

Special Note

- Any patient unconscious at the scene of a fire should be suspected of having carbon monoxide poisoning and treated accordingly.

Pediatric Note

- Aminophylline should be used with caution in children under 12 years of age.

Transport

- Use Code 3 if either laryngeal edema or laryngospasm is present.
- If carbon monoxide poisoning is suspected, use 100% oxygen and hyperventilate enroute.

SNAKEBITE

History

- How long ago was the patient bitten?
- When did the symptoms first appear?
- Where on the patient is the bite located?
- What kind of snake was it?
- Does the patient have shortness of breath, tingling around the mouth, abdominal cramps, chest pain, weakness, nausea, or muscle tremors?
- Has the patient's level of consciousness changed since the incident?
- Was any treatment instituted prior to the arrival of the paramedics?
- Is there any history of respiratory or cardiovascular disease?

Physical Exam

- Is the patient having any respiratory distress?
- What is the level of consciousness?
- Are there any fang marks?
- Is there more than one bite?
- Is there redness, pain, or swelling at the site?
- What are the vital signs?
- What is the skin temperature, color, and moisture?
- Are the lungs clear to auscultation?
- What is the EKG pattern?
- Are there any signs of systemic involvement?

Differential Diagnosis

- Must differentiate between local and systemic reaction.
- Must determine whether or not an allergic reaction is also present.

Treatment:

1. Administer high-flow oxygen if patient is having respiratory distress.
2. Lay the patient down and instruct him not to move unnecessarily.
3. Place a constricting band proximal to the site, if feasible, to occlude only venous return.
4. Keep area dependent to slow circulation of venom.
5. Apply cool pack to extremity; do *not* use ice in direct contact with skin and do *not* soak area in ice water.
6. Start an IV of D$_5$W TKO.
7. If the injury was less than 10 minutes ago and the hospital is more than an hour away, incise the site and apply constant suction:
   a. incisions must be *small,* from ⅛ to ¼ inch deep, ¼ inch long
   b. incise directly over the fang marks, keeping the incisions parallel to the extremity if possible.

Special Note

- Do not give analgesics.
- If the snake is dead, bring it in for positive identification.
- Might administer conjunctival skin test for antivenin sensitivity prior to arrival at the hospital.
- Not all bites of poisonous snakes actually inject venom.
- If reaction is severe, patient may suffer neurological abnormalities and/or cardiovascular collapse.

Pediatric Note

- Children will be more severely affected because of the proportionately large volume of venom injected.

Transport

- Transport promptly, as patient is in need of antivenin as soon as possible.
- Do not allow the patient to walk to the ambulance; must be carried and prevented from any unnecessary movement.
- All snakebite victims should be evaluated in the ED.

TRAUMA

History

- When did the injury occur?
- When did the symptoms begin?
- What was the mechanism of injury?
- Will extrication be required?
- Is there any blood loss; if so, what is the estimated volume?
- Does the patient have any pain; if so, where?
- Was the patient ever unconscious; if so, was it immediate with the injury or was there a lucid interval?
- Are there any underlying medical conditions?
- Is the patient on any medications?
- Has the patient injested any alcohol or drugs?

Physical Exam

- Is the respiratory system involved?
- What is the effectiveness of respirations?
- Is there any major controllable bleeding?
- What is the level of consciousness?
- Are there any systemic signs of shock?
- What are the vital signs?
- What does the EKG show?
- What are the findings of a head-to-toe exam?
- What is the status of circulatory and neurological function in the involved body part?

Differential Diagnosis

- Identify specific injuries and set priorities for treatment (flail chest, aortic tear, ruptured spleen, penetrating abdominal wound).
- Minor trauma may progress to major if not managed effectively.
- Look for any underlying medical conditions that may have precipitated the accident (seizure, heart).

Treatment

1. Assure the airway while keeping the spine immobilized; provide ventilatory assistance if necessary.
2. Give high-flow oxygen.
3. Control active bleeding.
4. Start an IV of RL or NS, using a large bore cannula needle and run to maintain blood pressure; may need to start more than one IV.
5. Apply antishock trousers if indicated.
6. Keep patient warm.
7. Do not give analgesics or oral fluids.
8. Apply dressings as needed.
9. Splint any fractures; immobilize spine as indicated.

Special Note

- If fluid replacement isn't effective and the antishock trousers are not working or are contraindicated, may try volume expanders, dopamine, or vasopressors.
- If extreme pain is contributing to shock and patient is trapped and cannot be extricated for some time, morphine sulfate might be given in 2–mg increments IV push.
- If injury is isolated, such as a hand caught in machinery, may consider morphine sulfate in 2–mg increments for pain.
- Trauma can be classified as minor because it affects a small part of the body, but still require urgent, or

sophisticated care depending on the body part affected, e.g., hand, eye, or neck.

Pediatric Note

Index of suspicion for child abuse includes:
- History of repeated injuries, ingestions, non-substantiated complaints, and/or delay in seeking care
- Discrepancy between history and injury
- Third party blamed for injuries (especially siblings)
- Alleged self-injury of an infant

If child abuse is suspected, be nonjudgmental at the scene and relay your suspicions to the physician privately once you arrive at the hospital.

Transport

- No need for Code 3 if patient is stabilized.
- Stabilize all injuries before moving the patient.
- With multisystem injuries, *do not* delay in the field; transport immediately and institute treatment enroute.

TRIAGE

History

- What type of emergency is this?
- Are environmental conditions presenting danger to patients or rescuers?
- How many patients are involved?
- What kind of manpower is available; have you called for backup?
- Are ambulances available at the scene?
- Which patients need immediate transport?

Physical Exam

Following the initial triage survey of all patients:
- How many patients require priority care (respiratory

distress, active bleeding, altered level of consciousness, head injury, or multiple injuries)?

- How many patients do not require priority treatment?
- How many patients are obviously dead or unresuscitatable with available manpower?

Following secondary survey of individual patients in order of priority:

- Is the respiratory system involved (trauma to the face, trachea, or chest)?
- Is there any major controllable bleeding?
- Are there any signs of shock (pulse, skin, level of consciousness)?
- What injuries are identified on brief head–to–toe exam?
- Is more extensive assessment indicated (repeat vital signs, neurological exam, EKG)?

Differential Diagnosis

- Don't overlook the possibility of underlying medical conditions.

Treatment

Each patient is treated in order of priority; scope of treatment is modified according to available manpower and resources.

1. Open the airway, assist ventilations if necessary, and give oxygen.
2. Control any active bleeding.
3. Immobilize spine and splint fractures.
4. Apply antishock trousers if indicated.
5. Keep patient warm.
6. Start an IV with a large bore needle; administer RL, NS, or volume expanders to maintain blood pressure.
7. Reassess frequently.
8. Do not give analgesics or oral fluids.

Special Note

- The role of the paramedic in a multiple casualty incident is primarily sophisticated assessment, direction of patient management, and basic life support. Advanced life support is only appropriate if there is a small number of patients.

Transport

- Transport patients as soon as ambulances are available; do not delay at the scene.
- Load ambulances according to patient problem and severity; direct ambulances to appropriate hospitals according to specialized care capabilities as well as even patient distribution.

PHARMACOLOGY:

EMERGENCY DRUGS

INTRODUCTION

This section contains individual profiles on a wide range of medications commonly used by paramedics in the United States and those generally carried on emergency vehicles.* The dosages used in this handbook conform to current standards for Advanced Cardiac Life Support as designated by the American Heart Association.

Although the specific drugs, dosages, routes, and indications may vary in your particular area, we have made an attempt to provide a rapid but complete review of these medications with emphasis on their pre-hospital application. These drug profiles are not intended to teach all there is to know about the pharmacological agents you carry but are intended to supplement and reinforce your present knowledge.

Remember that these medications are potent chemicals that can cause patient deterioration or even death if used improperly. You must have a thorough knowledge of all the medications you carry to avoid errors in administration. The actions, dosages, routes, indications, side effects, and other pertinent information should be committed to memory. Each time you receive a drug order, review your knowledge of the drug to be sure it is being administered properly. Question all orders that you are unsure of, and don't hesitate to question or even refuse an order if you feel it would be detrimental to the patient.

A section has been included on drugs commonly found in the home. This reference is indexed to provide ready information on the indications and actions of drugs which the emergency patient may be taking on a daily basis.

For greater accuracy, pediatric drug dosages are always calculated by the child's weight in kilograms. When calculating pediatric drug dosages, remember that the pediatric dose should never exceed the adult dose range.

---

*This listing does not purport to be an endorsement by the authors of any of the drugs mentioned herein.

Aminophylline

Theophylline

CLASS:	bronchodilator (smooth muscle relaxant)

USES:
- asthma
- congestive heart failure and pulmonary edema with associated cardiac asthma

ACTION:
- relaxes involuntary muscles and relieves bronchospasm
- increases heart rate and cardiac output
- stimulates respiratory drive
- decreases venous pressure by vasodilatation
- acts as a mild diuretic

DOSAGE/ ROUTE: 250–500 mg (2–5 mg/kg) in 20 cc D_5W (Volutrol) over 20–30 minutes per IV drip

SIDE EFFECTS:
- arrhythmias (PVCs, PACs, and tachycardias)
- hypotension
- convulsions

CONTRA– INDICATIONS:
- use with caution in children under age 12
- hypotension

SPECIAL INFORMATION:
- If infused too rapidly, it may cause arrhythmias, ventricular fibrillation, and/or circulatory collapse.
- Side effects occur more frequently with a hypoxic patient.
- Check lung sounds for effectiveness of the drug.
- Monitor EKG.
- Check blood pressure frequently.

PEDIATRIC DOSAGE: Epinephrine is drug of choice.

Ammonia Ampules

Ammonia Inhalant, Aromatic Spirit

CLASS: respiratory stimulant

USES:
- syncope
- to determine level of consciousness

ACTION: Inhalation of vapors irritates the mucous membranes of the upper respiratory system. This stimulates the respiratory and vasomotor centers of the medulla, causing an increase in respiration and blood pressure.

DOSAGE/ ROUTE: 2–3 inhalations

SIDE EFFECTS: none expected with normal use

CONTRA– INDICATIONS: Use with caution in patients with chronic obstructive pulmonary disease (COPD) or asthma—may cause bronchospasm.

SPECIAL INFORMATION: Be sure patient has inhaled sufficient vapor to elicit a response.

Aramine

Metaraminol Bitartrate

CLASS: vasopressor

USES: hypotensive states

ACTION:
- peripheral vasoconstrictor—less potent and longer lasting than Levophed
- increases force of myocardial contraction

DOSAGE/ ROUTE:

IV push	IV drip
0.5 mg *slowly*— may repeat one time in 15 min	100–200 mg in 250–500 cc D_5W— titrate to blood pressure

150

**SIDE
EFFECTS:**

- hypertension
- arrhythmias—tachycardia, bradycardia, and ventricular irritability

**CONTRA–
INDICATIONS:**

- hypovolemia, until fluid replacement is instituted

**SPECIAL
INFORMATION:** Start IV drip at *low* infusion rate and increase *gradually* to prevent hypertension and cardiac arrest.
Tissue necrosis may occur with infiltration—discontinue IV drip, circle area of infiltration, and report to base hospital.

**PEDIATRIC
DOSAGE:**

IV Push	IV Drip
0.01 mg/kg	50-100 mg. in 250 ml D₅W 0.4 mg/kg

Atropine Sulfate

Cardiac

CLASS: parasympathetic blocker

USES:

- bradycardias
- heart blocks

ACTION:

- blocks the action of the vagus nerve
- increases SA node conduction
- increases AV node conduction
- produces generalized sympathetic effect

**DOSAGE/
ROUTE:** 0.5–1.0 mg IV push

**SIDE
EFFECTS:**

- dries mucous membranes
- causes pupillary dilatation
- toxicity:
  flushed, warm, dry skin; dry mucous membranes; restlessness; decreased level of consciousness; irritability; hallucinations

151

CONTRA–
INDICATIONS: to be used with caution in:
- MI patient (may increase infarct size)
- glaucoma patient (increases intraocular pressure)

SPECIAL
INFORMATION: may suppress PVCs seen in a sinus brady-cardia by overriding the irritable ectopic focus

PEDIATRIC
DOSAGE: 0.01–0.02 mg/kg/dose IV push

Atropine Sulfate

Organophosphate Poisoning

CLASS: parasympathetic blocker

USES: organophosphate poisoning

ACTION: competes with acetylcholine for receptor sites at the synapse, thus blocking the para-sympathetic response to organophosphate
- increases SA node conduction
- increases AV node conduction
- decreases secretions
- produces generalized sympathetic effects by reduction of parasympathetic tone

DOSAGE/
ROUTE:
- 2 mg IV push or IM
- may repeat every 3–8 minutes as needed

SIDE
EFFECTS: toxicity:
flushed, warm, dry skin; dry mucous mem-branes; restlessness; decreased level of con-sciousness; irritability; hallucinations

CONTRA–
INDICATIONS: none in organophosphate poisoning

SPECIAL
INFORMATION:
- Monitor EKG closely.
- Effectiveness of atropine is determined by a

decrease in secretions and an increase of
heart rate if bradycardia is present.
- Atropine will not reverse the muscle weakness associated with organophosphate poisoning—the drug PAM (Protopam) is used for this purpose.

**PEDIATRIC
DOSAGE:**   0.05 mg/kg/dose IV push or IM
may repeat every 3–8 minutes as needed

Benadryl

Diphenhydramine

CLASS: antihistamine

USES:
- severe allergic reactions
- anaphylaxis (Note: drug of choice is epinephrine)

ACTION:
- binds to histamine receptor sites, thus suppressing allergic reaction
- has an associated sedative effect

**DOSAGE/
ROUTE:**   25–50 mg *slow* IV push or deep IM

**SIDE
EFFECTS:**
- decreases level of consciousness
- decreases blood pressure
- Overdose can lead to convulsions, coma, and death.
- thickens bronchial secretions due to its drying effect

**CONTRA–
INDICATIONS:**
- asthma attacks
- presence of alcohol and/or other depressant drugs

**PEDIATRIC
DOSAGE:**   2–5 mg/kg/dose *slow* IV push or IM

Calcium Chloride, 10%

CaCl$_2$

CLASS:	electrolyte

USES:
- asystole
- fine ventricular fibrillation
- electromechanical dissociation (e.g., idioventricular rhythm)

ACTION: increases myocardial contractility

DOSAGE/ ROUTE: 250–500 mg *slow* IV push or IC

SIDE EFFECTS: rare when given as recommended

CONTRA– INDICATIONS: use with caution in patients taking Lanoxin.

SPECIAL INFORMATION:
- given after $NaHCO_3$ and epinephrine have been administered
- precipitates if mixed with $NaHCO_3$
- potent local irritant
- given at a slow steady rate IV push to prevent clotting

PEDIATRIC DOSAGE: IV push—maximum dose of 20 mg/kg
IC—1.0 ml/5 kg diluted 1:1 with saline

Dextrose, 50%

D$_{50}$W, 50% Glucose

CLASS: carbohydrate

USES:
- hypoglycemia
- unconscious diabetic
- diagnostic tool in coma or seizures of unknown etiology

ACTION: quick release of sugar into blood for metabolism

**DOSAGE/
ROUTE:** 25 gm IV push (direct or through IV line)

**SIDE
EFFECTS:** tissue necrosis if infiltration occurs

**CONTRA–
INDICATIONS:** none for field use

**SPECIAL
INFORMATION:** • Always draw blood sugar prior to administration of 50% dextrose—label with patient's
name, date, and "pre-dextrose."
• Avoid IM or SQ routes.
• Make sure injection is intravenous; aspirate
before and during injection to insure you are
still in the vein.
• One bolus of 50% dextrose will not significantly increase the blood sugar level in a hyperglycemic patient.

**PEDIATRIC
DOSAGE:** 0.5–1 gm/kg slow IV push (25% solution)

Epinephrine 1:10,000

Adrenalin, "Epi"

CLASS: natural catecholamine (both alpha and beta
properties)

USES: • severe cardiac arrhythmia as in asystole or
in idioventricular rhythm
• in fine ventricular fibrillation to increase the
success of counter shock
• severe anaphylaxis

ACTION: Beta effects:
• increases heart rate
• increases cardiac output
• increases AV conduction
• increases irritability
• produces secondary bronchodilatation
Alpha effects:
• peripheral vasoconstriction

155

**DOSAGE/
ROUTE:**   0.5–1 mg 1:10,000 IV push, IC, or via ET tube

**SIDE
EFFECTS:**   tachyarrhythmias (supraventricular and ventricular)

**CONTRA–
INDICATIONS:** none for field use

**SPECIAL
INFORMATION:**
- If preloads aren't available, an ampule of 1:1000 (1 mg/cc) can be diluted with 9 cc of normal saline to equal 1:10,000/10 cc.
- Monitor EKG and peripheral pulses for effectiveness.

**PEDIATRIC
DOSAGE:**   0.1 mg/kg 1:10,000 IV push or IC

Epinephrine 1:1000

Adrenalin, "Epi"

CLASS: natural catecholamine

USES:
- bronchial asthma
- anaphylaxis

ACTION: Beta effects:
- reduces bronchospasm by relaxing smooth muscles in the bronchial tree (bronchodilatation)
- secondary cardiotonic effects

Alpha effects:
- peripheral vasoconstriction

**DOSAGE/
ROUTE:**   0.3 mg 1:1000 SQ—may repeat 3 times at 5-minute intervals

**SIDE
EFFECTS:**   Major:
tachyarrhythmias (supraventricular and ventricular)
Minor:
pallor, cool skin

CONTRA–
INDICATIONS:
- Use with caution in pregnancy—decreases placental blood flow and can induce early labor.
- Use with caution in patients with preexisting tachycardias.

SPECIAL
INFORMATION:
- If severe anaphylaxis, may give 0.1 mg SQ at site of sting (do not inject fingers or toes).
- Monitor EKG, vital signs, and lung sounds frequently.
- Be prepared to give epinephrine 1:10,000 IV push for circulatory collapse/cardiac arrest.

PEDIATRIC
DOSAGE:
0.1 mg 1:1000 SQ—may repeat 3 times at 20-min intervals

Glucola

Carbonated Carbohydrate Solution, Glucose Solution

CLASS: carbohydrate

USES: *alert* hypoglycemic patient

ACTION: provides free sugar for quick absorption into the blood stream

DOSAGE/
ROUTE: 210 ml (75 gm) orally

SIDE
EFFECTS: none if used as directed

CONTRA–
INDICATIONS: patients with an absent gag reflex or decreased level of consciousness who are unable to drink without assistance

SPECIAL
INFORMATION:
- Always draw blood sugar prior to administration of glucola—label with patient's name, date, and "pre-glucola."

- Check for presence of gag reflex prior to administration

PEDIATRIC DOSAGE: 30–210 ml, varies depending upon child's weight

Inderal

Propranolol

CLASS: antiarrhythmic: beta blocker

USES: supraventricular tachycardias*

ACTION:
- inhibits the adrenergic response by blocking the beta receptors within the myocardium
- decreases AV conduction
- decreases heart rate and contractility, thereby reducing myocardial oxygen consumption and workload
- suppresses atrial and ventricular ectopics

DOSAGE/ ROUTE: 1–4 mg slow IV push—0.5 mg increments every 1 min until desired effect is achieved

SIDE EFFECTS:
- bradycardia and heart blocks
- hypotension
- may precipitate congestive heart failure due to decrease in contractility
- may cause bronchospasm in patients with asthma

CONTRA– INDICATIONS: Use with caution in:
- asthmatics
- congestive heart failure *not* precipitated by tachyarrhythmias
- pregnancy
- patients on antihypertensive or diuretic drugs

---

*Usually tried after Valsalva maneuver and/or carotid sinus massage.

SPECIAL INFORMATION:
- Monitor patient closely while administering and watch for arrhythmias.
- Inderal (10–40 mg) orally is a common home medication for the treatment of severe coronary insufficiency (angina).

PEDIATRIC DOSAGE:
- rarely used; given in 0.5 mg increments, not to exceed 0.1 mg/kg/dose every 15 minutes
- total dose should not exceed 2 mg

Instant Glucose Paste

CLASS: carbohydrate

USES: hypoglycemic patients (alert or nonalert), when no IV line can be established

ACTION: quick source of free glucose for body metabolism

DOSAGE/ ROUTE:
- 12.5 gm (½ tube) between cheek and teeth
- may repeat

SIDE EFFECTS: none for field use

CONTRA– INDICATIONS: none

SPECIAL INFORMATION:
- Draw blood sugar first if possible.
- Watch airway if patient is comatose, prevent aspiration.
- Position patient on side with medication in dependent cheek.

PEDIATRIC DOSAGE:
- 12.5 gm (½ tube) between cheek and teeth
- may repeat

Intropin

Dopamine, Dopamine Hydrochloride

CLASS: natural catecholamine (both alpha and beta properties)

USES: Shock
- cardiogenic (drug of choice)
- low resistance (septic, anaphylactic)
- hypovolemic (after sufficient volume replacement)

ACTION:
- increases cardiac output by increasing contractility and stroke volume, thereby increasing blood pressure
- selectively dilates blood vessels supplying the brain, kidneys, heart, and gastrointestinal tract
- heart rate increases slightly or not at all
- significant alpha effect *only* in very large doses

DOSAGE/ ROUTE:
- 400–800 mg/250–500 cc D_5W IV drip (titrate to blood pressure)
- suggested drip rates:
  start at 10 μgtt/minute for moderate hypotension
  start at 20 μgtt/minute for severe hypotension

SIDE EFFECTS:
- ventricular irritability (occurs less frequently than with Isuprel)
- nausea, vomiting, and angina (rarely)
- hypertension and extreme vasoconstriction can occur with high infusion rates.
- hypotension can occur with low infusion

CONTRA– INDICATIONS: none for field use

**SPECIAL
INFORMATION:**
- Base hospital should give drip rate with order.
- Titrate to blood pressure and patient response.
- Ask base hospital where to maintain blood pressure (check every 5–10 min).
- Tissue necrosis may occur with infiltration
    discontinue IV drip
    circle area of infiltration and inform base hospital
- Approximately 10 minutes after drip is stopped, effects of the drug cease.
- Don't mix with an IV solution of sodium bicarbonate.

**PEDIATRIC
DOSAGE:**

Use 200 mg in 500 cc D_5W (concentration of 400 μgm/ml). Begin with 5 μg/kg/min, titrating to blood pressure.

Ipecac

Syrup of Ipecac

CLASS: emetic

USES: overdose in *alert* patient

ACTION:
- irritates lining of stomach
- stimulates vomiting center in the medulla—onset within 20–30 minutes

**DOSAGE
ROUTE:**   30 ml orally, may repeat in 30 minutes

**SIDE
EFFECTS:**   none

**CONTRA–
INDICATIONS:**
- ingested petroleum distillates
- caustic agents
- unknown agents

**SPECIAL
INFORMATION:**
- Check for presence of gag reflex prior to administration.
- Watch level of consciousness and airway after administration until emesis occurs.
- Accompany with large amounts of water or clear fluids to dilute.
- Save emesis for analysis.

**PEDIATRIC
DOSAGE:**
15 ml child (1 tablespoon)
30 ml adolescent (2 tablespoons)

Isuprel

Isoproterenol Hydrochloride (1:5000)

CLASS: synthetic catecholamine (pure beta)

USES:
- severe bradycardias
- AV blocks refractory to Atropine
- idioventricular rhythms

ACTION:
- increases heart rate
- increases cardiac output
- speeds SA, AV, and ventricular conduction
- increases myocardial oxygen consumption
- produces secondary bronchodilatation and peripheral vasodilatation

**DOSAGE/
ROUTE:**
1–2 mg/250–500 cc D_5W IV drip titrated to pulse

**SIDE
EFFECTS:**
ventricular arrhythmias, tachycardias, and hypotension

**CONTRA–
INDICATIONS:** Use with caution in patients with acute MI.

**SPECIAL
INFORMATION:**
- Monitor EKG closely.
- Ask base hospital where pulse should be maintained.
- Check pulse and BP frequently.
- Isuprel has cumulative effects when used with epinephrine.

**PEDIATRIC
DOSAGE:** 1 mg in 250 cc D₅W titrated to pulse

Isuprel Mistometer

Isoproterenol Hydrochloride (1:400)

CLASS:
- bronchodilator
- synthetic catecholamine (pure beta)

USES: asthma attacks

ACTION:
- dilates bronchioles by relaxing smooth muscles
- secondary cardiotonic effects (see Isuprel)

**DOSAGE/
ROUTE:**
- 1–2 deep inhalations, may repeat once after 5 minutes
- Have patient hold inhalation for a few seconds before exhaling.

**SIDE
EFFECTS:** ventricular arrhythmias, tachycardias

**CONTRA–
INDICATIONS:** preexisting tachyarrhythmias from prior use of drug

**SPECIAL
INFORMATION:**
- Check lung sounds before and after administration to determine effectiveness of drug.
- If no effect try epinephrine and/or Aminophylline.
- Report to base hospital any use of antiasthmatic drugs prior to your arrival (patients frequently overuse their Mistometers

and may develop paradoxic bronchocon-
striction).
- Monitor EKG.

**PEDIATRIC
DOSAGE:** rarely used

Lanoxin

Digoxin, "Dig"

CLASS: cardiotonic

USES:
- supraventricular tachycardias
- congestive heart failure

ACTION: improves stroke volume and cardiac output
and lowers myocardial oxygen consumption
by:
- increasing strength of myocardial contraction
- slowing conduction at the SA and AV nodes

**DOSAGE/
ROUTE:** 0.25–0.5 mg IV push

**SIDE
EFFECTS:** bradycardias or AV blocks
toxicity:
- GI disturbances
- visual disturbances
- arrhythmias—ventricular bigeminy, PAT
with block, sinus arrest

**CONTRA–
INDICATIONS:** digitalis toxicity

**SPECIAL
INFORMATION:**
- Use caution when administering $CaCl_2$ or
cardioverting a patient who has received
Lanoxin.
- Patients with superventricular tachycardias
may be dig-toxic so elicit a thorough history
before treatment.

**PEDIATRIC
DOSAGE:** Should not be given to children in the field

Lasix

Furosemide

CLASS: diuretic

USES:
- congestive heart failure
- acute pulmonary edema

ACTION:
- acts on the kidneys to excrete water, sodium chloride, and potassium, which leads to a decreased circulating blood volume
- vasodilatation
- very potent with rapid onset—5–10 minutes

**DOSAGE/
ROUTE:**   20–80 mg IV push (up to 200 mg in *rare* field cases)

**SIDE
EFFECTS:**   none for field use

**CONTRA–
INDICATIONS:**
- Use with caution if patient is allergic to sulfonamides.
- children under 12 years of age
- pregnancy

**SPECIAL
INFORMATION:**
- Generally very safe acutely, but prolonged use or large doses can lead to potassium loss with dehydration, hypotension, and cardiac arrhythmias.
- Check to see if patient is on diuretics—may need a larger dose to reach the desired effect.
- Check lung sounds before and after administration to determine effectiveness of drug.

**PEDIATRIC
DOSAGE:**   not used

Levophed

Levarterenol Bitartrate, Norepinephrine

CLASS:
- natural catecholamine (mostly alpha)
- vasopressor

USES: hypotensive states

ACTION:
- potent vasoconstrictor which increases blood pressure by direct effect on peripheral blood vessels
- dilates coronary arteries

DOSAGE/ ROUTE: 1–2 ampules (4–8 mg) in 250–500 cc D_5W IV drip—titrate to blood pressure*

SIDE EFFECTS:
- severe hypertension
- bradycardia

CONTRA– INDICATIONS: hypovolemia until fluid replacement is instituted

SPECIAL INFORMATION:
- Tissue necrosis will occur with infiltration.
- Discontinue IV drip, circle area of infiltration, and inform base hospital.
- Increased blood pressure may stimulate baroreceptors, causing a reflex bradycardia; may need to use atropine.
- Monitor perfusion parameters—quality of pulses, skin color, temperature, and level of consciousness.

PEDIATRIC DOSAGES: 2–4 mg in 250–500 ml D_5W IV drip–titrate to blood pressure

---

*Maintain blood pressure between 90–100 systolic.

Mannitol

CLASS:	osmotic diuretic; cellular dehydrating agent
USES:	head injury with signs of increased intracranial pressure
ACTION:	• draws fluid from brain cells and intracellular spaces • promotes urine flow
DOSAGE/ ROUTE:	250 mg/kg IV drip per Volutrol over 5 minutes
SIDE EFFECTS:	renal failure
CONTRA– INDICATIONS:	• suspected intracranial hemorrhage • hypersensitivity • severe renal failure • congestive heart failure • use with caution in hypovolemia and pregnancy

SPECIAL INFORMATION:	• If crystals are seen in the solution *do not* use it.
	• Use inline filter for administration.
	• Monitor vital and neurologic signs closely.
	• Signs of increased intracranial pressure include:
	    decreased level of consciousness
	    hypertension
	    bradycardia
	    abnormal respiratory pattern
	    pupil changes

PEDIATRIC DOSAGE:	250 mg/kg IV drip per Volutrol over 5 minutes

Morphine Sulfate

M.S., MSO$_4$

CLASS:	• narcotic • analgesic

USES:	• acute myocardial infarction
	• acute pulmonary edema
	• burns
	• isolated injuries

ACTION:
- decreases pain perception and anxiety
- relaxes respiratory effort
- causes peripheral vasodilatation, thereby decreasing the blood return to the heart (pharmacologic rotating tourniquets)

DOSAGE/ ROUTE:

IV push	IM
2–15 mg in 2 mg increments every 1–2 minutes (titrate to effect)	5–15 mg based on patient's weight

SIDE EFFECTS:

Major: respiratory depression and/or arrest
Minor: decreased level of consciousness
transient hypotension

CONTRA– INDICATIONS:
- head injury
- undiagnosed abdominal pain
- multiple trauma
- use with caution in chronic lung disease or compromised respirations

SPECIAL INFORMATION: Narcan will reverse overdose effects.

PEDIATRIC DOSAGE: 0.1–0.2 mg/kg IV push

Narcan

Naloxone

CLASS: narcotic antagonist

USES:
- nonalert narcotic overdose
- diagnostic tool in coma of unknown origin

ACTION: reverses respiratory depression as well as other effects of narcotic overdose by de-activating the narcotic

**DOSAGE/
ROUTE:**

- 0.4–0.8 mg (1–2 ampules) IV push, IM, or sublingual
- Patient may not respond to initial dosage; may have to repeat dose up to 10–15 times in order to elicit an adequate response.

**SIDE
EFFECTS:**

none (even in the absence of a narcotic)

**CONTRA–
INDICATIONS:**

**SPECIAL
INFORMATION:**

- Quick onset of action (30 seconds to 2 minutes).
- Onset of action for IM dose is within 2 minutes.
- Short-acting drug: may repeat as necessary while narcotic is still in the patient's system. Watch for a relapse with respiratory depression and coma.
- Narcan can precipitate withdrawal syndrome and/or combative behavior in addicts.
- Narcan has no pharmacologic effect if narcotic is not present in the system.
- Do not insert esophageal airway prior to administration of Narcan.
- Effective against natural and synthetic narcotics:

Codeine	Lomotil
Darvon	Methadone
Demerol	Morphine
Dilaudid	Paregoric
Heroin	Percodan

**PEDIATRIC
DOSAGE:**

0.005 mg/kg IV push, IM, or sublingual—may repeat as necessary

Nitroglycerin

NTG, TNT, Nitro

CLASS: vasodilator

USES: angina pectoris

ACTION: a systemic vasodilator which decreases right heart return by venous "pooling," therefore decreasing myocardial workload and oxygen consumption

**DOSAGE/
ROUTE:**
- 1 tablet 0.4 mg (1/150 gr) sublingual
- may repeat

**SIDE
EFFECTS:**
- decrease in blood pressure
- temporary pulsating headache and facial flushing

**CONTRA–
INDICATIONS:**
- hypotension
- children under 12 years of age
- use with caution in the presence of prolonged acute chest pain

**SPECIAL
INFORMATION:**
- Always check blood pressure before and after administration.
- Tablets should be stored in a dark place to maintain potency.
- Tablets taste bitter and sting when placed under the tongue (if bitter taste is absent suspect outdated drug).
- Nitroglycerine is a very unstable drug. Once bottle has been opened, it should be replaced in 30 days.

**PEDIATRIC
DOSAGE:**   not used in children

Physostigmine Salicylate

ESERINE SALICYLATE

CLASS: cholinergic

USES: antidote for symptomatic overdose of tricyclic antidepressants and belladonna alkaloids

ACTION: promotes increase in acetylcholine by inhibiting cholinesterase activity

DOSAGE/ ROUTE:
- 2 mg in 10 cc IV Volutrol over 2 minutes
- may repeat twice at 5-minute intervals
- maximum dosage 6 mg

SIDE EFFECTS
- bradycardia
- excessive lacrimation, salivation and sweating
- increased GI motility
- seizures
- urinary incontinence

CONTRA– INDICATIONS:
- asthma and COPD
- cardiovascular disease
- bradyarrhythmias

SPECIAL INFORMATION:
- Toxic symptoms may be reversed by atropine
- Watch for respiratory difficulty, bronchospasm and laryngospasm.
- Have suction equipment available to control secretions.
- Repeat dosages are dependent on amount of drug ingested.
- Seizures may occur if given too rapidly.
- Effectiveness of Physostigmine is determined by 1) slowing of heart rate, 2) improvement in level of consciousness, and 3) return of moist mucous membranes.
- Some common tricyclic antidepressants are Elavil, Triavil, Tofranil, Sinequan, Aventyl, and Vivactil

171

- Some common belladonna alkaloids are atropine, scopolamine, hyoscine, hyoscyamine, and Jimson weed

PEDIATRIC DOSAGES:
- 0.5–2 mg in 10 cc IV Volutrol over 2 min
- may repeat twice at 5-min intervals
- limit use to life-threatening situations

Pitocin

Oxytocin

CLASS: oxytocic

USES: postpartum hemorrhage

ACTION: constricts uterine musculature, thereby causing constriction of uterine blood vessels

DOSAGE/ ROUTE:

IM	IV drip
3–10 units	10–20 units of 500–1000 cc D_5W or Ringer's lactate Titrate to severity of hemorrhage and uterine response

SIDE EFFECTS:
- anaphylaxis
- cardiac arrhythmias

CONTRA– INDICATIONS: Only used *after* delivery of the infant and placenta.
Use with extreme caution in patients with previous Cesarean section or uterine surgery.

SPECIAL INFORMATION:
- If administered prior to delivery of infant and placenta, uterus may rupture with subsequent maternal and infant death.
- Uterine effect occurs within 1 minute and

lasts up to 30 minutes after the infusion is discontinued.
- To be used in conjunction with other methods of postpartum hemorrhage control such as fluid replacement, uterine massage, baby to breast, shock position.

Sodium Bicarbonate
"Bicarb," $NaHCO_3$

CLASS:	alkalotic agent (base)
USES:	to combat acidosis in respiratory or cardiac arrest
ACTION:	reduces acidosis by direct release of base radicals into the bloodstream
DOSAGE/ ROUTE:	1 mEq/kg for first two doses—subsequent dosages of 0.5 mEq/kg dependent on respiratory status
SIDE EFFECTS:	alkalosis if given too frequently in a patient being well ventilated
CONTRA– INDICATIONS:	none
SPECIAL INFORMATION:	Precipitates if mixed with calcium chloride.
PEDIATRIC DOSAGE:	1 mEq/kg IV push

Valium
Diazepam

CLASS:	• anticonvulsant • sedative
USES:	• sustained and/or recurrent grand mal seizures

- precardioversion
- acute stress reaction (rarely)

ACTION:
- decreases cerebral irritability
- relaxes skeletal muscles

DOSAGE/ ROUTE:
- IV push in increments of 2.5 mg over 1 min, titrated to effect
- usual range 2.5–20 mg
- can give up to 40 mg with status epilepticus
- 5–10 mg can be given IM

SIDE EFFECTS:
Major: respiratory depression or arrest
Minor: drowsiness, vertigo, ataxia, transient hypotension

CONTRA– INDICATIONS:
Use with caution in:
- shock states
- children under 12 years of age
- pregnant women

SPECIAL INFORMATION:
- Causes respiratory arrest if given too fast or too much—never give without resuscitation equipment available to assist ventilation if necessary.
- Do not mix or dilute with another drug or IV solution because it precipitates.
- When giving IV push, inject as close to needle as possible to prevent precipitation in tubing.
- Is very painful upon administration.
- Has a cumulative effect with alcohol and sedatives.

PEDIATRIC DOSAGE:
0.05 mg/kg/dose slow IV push, to maximum of 10 mg—titrating to seizure

Xylocaine

Lidocaine Hydrochloride, 2%

CLASS: antiarrhythmic

USES:
- ventricular irritability
- intractable ventricular fibrillation
- prophylactically in the presence of chest pain

ACTION: decreases ventricular excitability without depressing the force of ventricular contractions

DOSAGE/ ROUTE:

IV bolus	IV drip
50–100 mg	1–2 gm in 250–500 cc D_5W

Maximum dosage is 4 mg/kg/hr

SIDE EFFECTS: toxicity:
  Early: anxiety, euphoria, combativeness, nausea, twitchings, numbness
  Late: convulsions, decreased blood pressure, coma, widening of QRS complex, prolonged PR interval

CONTRA– INDICATIONS: Use with caution in:
- AV blocks
- sensitivity to lidocaine
- idioventricular or escape rhythms

SPECIAL INFORMATION:
- Onset of action after bolus is within 2 minutes and lasts approximately 10 to 20 minutes from the time bolus is given. Should be followed by a lidocaine drip
- May need to repeat a bolus if unable to start a lidocaine drip immediately
- In concentration of 2 gm in 500 cc it is usual to start IV drip at 1–2 mg/minute
- Concentration of 2 gm/500 cc D_5W
  1 mg/minute = 15 μgtt/min
  2 mg/minute = 30 μgtt/min
  3 mg/minute = 45 μgtt/min
  4 mg/minute = 60 μgtt/min

- Include frequency of PVC's when reporting EKG to base hospital.
- Decrease drip rate and inform base hospital at first indication of toxicity.

PEDIATRIC.
DOSAGE: 0.5–1 mg/kg/dose IV push to maximum of 50 mg/dose every 20 minutes

Dextrose, 5% in Water

5% DW, D$_5$W, 5DW

CLASS: crystalloid

USES:
- life-line for administration of medications
- mainly used to keep open IV
- for dilution of IV drip drugs

ACTION: glucose solution used for parenteral therapy

DOSAGE/
ROUTE: IV drip

SIDE
EFFECTS: Overhydration can occur if administered too rapidly.

CONTRA–
INDICATIONS: Use with caution in head injuries.

SPECIAL
INFORMATION: Content: 5% glucose in water, 50 gm dextrose/liter, (170 calories/liter)

Note: Whenever ordered to mix an IV drip medication (e.g., Isuprel), *always* piggyback it into a plain IV line of D$_5$W. In case you have to discontinue the medication, you will have a plain D$_5$W readily available.

PEDIATRIC
DOSAGE: IV drip, usually to keep open

Normal Saline

N.S., Saline, 0.9% Sodium Chloride Injection, Physiologic Saline, NaCl

CLASS:	crystalloid
USES:	• hypovolemia due to trauma • dehydration states (diabetic coma, heat exhaustion, etc.) • *irrigation* for eye injuries
ACTION:	• electrolyte solution which is osmotically equivalent to blood • increases circulating volume by remaining in the vascular system
DOSAGE/ ROUTE:	IV drip, regulated according to patient condition
SIDE EFFECTS:	overload may cause congestive heart failure
CONTRA– INDICATIONS:	• congestive heart failure • pulmonary edema
SPECIAL INFORMATION:	Content: 154 mEq Na/liter 154 mEq Cl/liter Do not mix with Valium
PEDIATRIC DOSAGE:	IV drip regulated according to body weight and patient status

Ringer's Lactate

Lactated Ringer's Solution, R/L

CLASS:	crystalloid
USES:	• hemorrhagic shock • fractures • multiple trauma • burns

177

- dehydration
- mild metabolic acidosis (diabetic keto-acidosis)

ACTION:
- approximates the electrolyte composition of blood and therefore increases circulating volume by remaining in the vascular system
- provides lactate for the correction of mild acidosis

DOSAGE/ ROUTE: IV drip rate dependent on patient status—may frequently be ordered to run Ringer's Lactate *wide open* with hypovolemic states

SIDE EFFECTS: Careful attention should be paid to vital signs and breath sounds so as not to overload patient. May need to decrease the infusion rate as patient condition improves.

CONTRA– INDICATIONS:
- Use with caution in patients with suspected congestive heart failure or head injuries.
- Contraindicated with severely impaired lactate metabolism such as occurs in liver disease or anoxic states (such as cardiac arrest).

SPECIAL INFORMATION:
- Content per liter:
  130 mEq Na
  109 mEq Cl
  4 mEq K
  3 mEq Ca
  28 mEq lactate
- Use large bore IV needle.

PEDIATRIC DOSAGE: dependent on weight and patient's status

Salt Poor Albumin

SPA Normal Serum Albumin, 25%

CLASS: colloid, plasma volume expander

Salt Poor Albumin

USES:
- severe shock states where the restoration of blood volume is urgent
- burns

ACTION:
- osmotic effect draws extravascular fluid into the circulatory system
- raises serum protein levels

DOSAGE/ ROUTE:
- 50 cc vial (12.5 gm albumin) IV drip, infuse as rapidly as possible
- may repeat as needed

SIDE EFFECTS:
- dyspnea
- pulmonary edema

CONTRA– INDICATIONS: Use with caution in cardiac failure.

SPECIAL INFORMATION:
- Content: a sterile natural plasma protein
- Do not use if the solution is cloudy.
- Check wounds after administration since bleeding may recur with an increase in blood pressure.

PEDIATRIC DOSAGE: dependent on weight and patient's status

PHARMACOLOGY:

COMMON HOME MEDICATIONS

INTRODUCTION

The variety of classes and actions of pharmacologic agents is so vast that a person would have to study for years to understand the complexities of the actions and uses of each. In the few short months of paramedic training, this obviously is impossible. You have learned in detail the properties and actions of the drugs you carry in your drug box; but what about the different kinds of medications that you as a paramedic will encounter daily in your field work?

Many times, the only clue you will have to the possible cause of the patient's problem will be a handful of prescription drugs found in the home. Sometimes the kinds of medications a person is taking will help to suggest a possible diagnosis. The following are categories of drugs commonly found in the home. Each summary gives a brief description of the uses and actions of these agents, as well as a sampling of some of the more common medications included in that category.

Analgesics

Analgesics are drugs that reduce pain. They can accomplish this in one or more of the following ways:
- raising the threshold of pain
- altering the psychologic response to pain
- alleviating anxiety and apprehension

The amount of pain a person experiences will vary from time to time depending on the patient's physical and emotional status, and will differ between individuals. Analgesics are not normally prescribed unless an attempt has been made to treat the cause of the pain, but often a patient is sent home on some type of analgesic to control pain during the treatment process. The type of analgesic ordered will depend largely on the cause of the pain, as well as on its location and severity. For clarity, these drugs have been divided here into *Mild Analgesics* and *Strong Analgesics*. The latter group includes both narcotic and nonnarcotic analgesics. Additionally, synthetic narcotics are considered *Strong Analgesics*.

Common Medications

Mild Analgesics:
  Aspirin (ASA)
  Aspirin, Phenacetin, and Caffeine (APCs, Bufferin)
  Darvon
  Darvon compound
  Tylenol (acetaminophen)
  Tylenol with codeine #3 (30 mg), #6 (60 mg)
Strong Analgesics
  Demerol
  Codeine
  Percodan
  Talwin
  Dilaudid
  Percogesic
  Cocaine
  Heroin
  Methadone
  Phenaphen

Anorexiants

Commonly called "diet pills," anorexiants are drugs that are given to control the appetite, usually to help the patient lose weight. The most common of these are the amphetamine or amphetamine-like drugs that have a tendency to produce psychic, and occasionally physical, dependency on the drug. Because of this side effect, most physicians now prefer to give nutritional guidance and psychologic counseling rather than prescribing these agents. The original explanation of the action of anorexiants suggested that they stimulate the central nervous system (CNS); this theory was discarded after recent studies showed that they actually affect the control center in the hypothalamus. These drugs will cause anorexia, but they also produce an increase in awareness, initiative, and motor activity, which contributes to a decreased sensation of fatigue.

Common Medications

Preludin
Tenuate (Tepanil)
Amphetamine (Benzedrine)
Dexadrine
Opatrol
Ritalin
Didrex
Pre–Sate
Plegine
Wilpo
Ionamin

Antacids

Antacids are agents used to reduce the acidity of the stomach and duodenum. They are particularly useful in controlling the symptoms of peptic ulcers, gastritis, indigestion, and other disorders of the upper gastrointestinal tract. By raising the pH of the stomach to 5.0, many of the adverse effects of hyperacidity can be greatly reduced.

Common Medications

Sodium bicarbonate
Maalox
Gelusil
Riopan
Amphojel
Mylanta

DiGel
PeptoBismol
Alka Seltzer

Antianginal Agents

Antianginal agents were originally labeled coronary vasodilators because they were thought to relieve angina by dilating coronary blood vessels. We now know that they also dilate the periphery to a small degree, thereby easing the workload of the heart and reducing the myocardial oxygen requirements.

Common Medications

Nitroglycerine
Isordil (sorbitrate)
Peritrate
Inderal (beta blocker)
Cardilate
Nitranitol
Amyl nitrate

Antiarrhythmics

As their name suggests, these agents are used to control the rhythm of the heart and prevent arrhythmias that could endanger the patient. These drugs are commonly prescribed following any kind of cardiac insult that would potentially produce rhythm disturbances. Such conditions include myocardial infarction, open heart surgery, pericarditis, congestive heart failure, and valvular disease.

Common Medications

Pronestyl (ventricular arrhythmias)
Quinidine (supraventricular & ventricular arrhythmias)
Inderal (supraventricular & ventricular arrhythmias)
Quinaglute (supraventricular & ventricular arrhythmias)
Dilantin (ventricular arrhythmias)

Antibiotics

Antibiotics are in widespread use to combat specific bacteria and other microorganisms once a culture is read to identify the cause. Certain strains of organisms become immune to the agents and require different drugs or dosing. Underdosing can result in recurrence of certain infections, while overdosing can result in severe diarrhea and nausea.

Common Medications

Penicillin
Erythromycin
Streptomycin
Ampicillin
Oxacillin
Dicloxacillin
Keflex
Tetracycline
Kantrex (kanamycin)
Nafcillin
Chloramphenicol

Anticoagulants

Anticoagulants act by prolonging the prothrombin time which produces a delay in blood clotting. These agents are essential in preventing thrombosis formation associated with various cardio-vascular diseases and following various cardiac and orthopedic operations. Patients sent home on oral anticoagulants are cautioned regarding the use of aspirin which can affect clotting. They are also instructed to watch for excessive bleeding and to have periodic laboratory studies to ensure they are on the right maintenance dose.

Common Medications

Coumadin (warfarin)
Dicumarol
Sintrom
Heparin for injection (rare)

Anticonvulsants

Anticonvulsant agents act by raising the threshold for cerebral irritation without greatly incapacitating the patient. The agents and the dosages are varied according to the type of seizures present and the patient status. They may be prescribed acutely or on a maintenance dose for life. Side effects and/or overdosing can inhibit fine motor coordination and therefore can limit the activities of those patients who require high doses for seizure control.

Common Medications

Dilantin } Principal home drug regimen
Phenobarbital } for seizure control
Mebaral
Mysoline
Mephenytoin (mesantoin)
Zarontin
Tridione

Antidepressants

A common psychiatric problem requiring drug therapy is depression. The two most common classifications of antidepressants currently in use have different pharmacologic actions. *Tricyclic compounds* potentiate the adrenergic effects by preventing the uptake of norepinephrine within the central nervous system. Severe tachyarrhythmias may occur from an overdose of these agents and may require Physostigmine or even defibrillation. *Monoamine oxidase (MAO) inhibitors* prevent impulse transmissions at the synapse between neurons and also may interrupt catecholamine breakdown. If the patient accidentally combines narcotics with MAO inhibitors or overdoses on MAO inhibitors, cardiac irritability may occur.

Common Medications

Tricyclic Compounds
  Tofranil
  Elavil
  Triavil
  Norpramin (Pertofrane)
  Adapin (Sinequan)
  Aventyl
  Vivactil
MAO Inhibitors
  Parnate
  Marplan
  Nardil

Antidiarrheal Agents

Diarrhea may occur either chronically or acutely as a result of various drugs, infections, allergies, or ischemic conditions. Specific agents which are used to restore the bowel's normal motility and absorption are listed below. Overdose of these drugs can result in paralytic ileus, with the patient complaining of severe abdominal pain.

Common Medications

Lomotil
Kaopectate
Paregoric
Donnagel PG
Bismuth salts
Furoxone
Bacid (Lactinex)
Flagyl
Kaolin with pectin
Parepectolin
Sorboquel

Antiemetic Agents

Antiemetic agents are indicated to prevent or relieve nausea and vomiting. These agents are very useful in patients with motion sickness or middle ear infections. Antiemetics are also used to counteract the nausea and vomiting which are caused by chemotherapy used to treat cancer patients. Oral preparations and rectal suppositories are often the prescribed routes of administration for home use. Drowsiness is a very common side effect of antiemetic agents because of their associated sedative action.

Common Medications

Compazine
Tigan
Dramamine
Phenergan

Thorazine
Trilafon } **phenothiazines**
Prolixin

Torecan

189

Antihistamines

Antihistamine agents help prevent further release of histamine in an allergic reaction, thus helping to suppress associated signs and symptoms. They are used for hay fever and urticaria but are of little value in preventing an acute asthma or allergic attack. Antihistamines have an associated sedative effect, so use in conjunction with alcohol or CNS depressants can cause a decreased level of consciousness or respiratory depression.

Common Medications

Benadryl
Chlor–Trimeton (Histaspan Teldrin)
Phenergan
Periactin
Dimetane
Disomer
Temaril
Pyrilamine maleate
Histadyl
Pyribenzamine citrate
Pribenzamine HCL
Decapryn
Clestin

Antihypertensive Agents

Antihypertensive agents are usually used in combination with other drugs such as diuretics and sedatives to lower and maintain the patient's blood pressure to a diastolic of 100 or below. Most antihypertensive drugs work by causing vasodilatation in the periphery. A common side effect of antihypertensive therapy is hypotension.

Common Medications

Serapes
Serpasil (Reserpine)
Apresoline
Aldomet (Methyldopa)
Diamox
Inversine
Ismelin

Antipsychotic Agents

Antipsychotic agents are major tranquilizers that are prescribed to alter the symptoms of acute and chronic behavioral disorders resulting from mental illness. In therapeutic doses, these medications enable the individual to cope with his/her illness and function in the activities of daily living, without producing the stuporous side effects of most sedatives. Since mental illness is a widespread affliction in today's society, you may encounter many patients on these medications.

Common Medications

Phenothiazine Agents:
   Thorazine
   Mellaril
   Trilafon
   Prolixin (Permitil)
   Quide
   Vesprin
   Serentil
   Tindal
   Stelazine
   Sparine
Thioxanthine Agents:
   Haldol
   Taractan
   Navane
   Indoklon
   Lithane (Eskalith, Lithonate)

Antispasmodics

Antispasmodics are used to relieve the pain associated with excessive gastrointestinal smooth muscle contractions. These agents are used in GI disorders such as colitis. They work by blocking acetylcholine in the parasympathetic nervous system. Antispasmodics very often produce associated central nervous system depression.

Common Medications

Pro-Banthine
Banthine
Donnatal
Belladonna extracts

Antituberculosis Agents

During the last 25 years there has been a sharp decline in the incidence of tuberculosis due to the use of chemotherapeutic agents. Antituberculosis drugs work against this inflammatory, communicable disease by deactivating the tubercle bacillus. Tuberculosis commonly attacks the lungs but may be found in any part of the body.

The drugs listed are frequently used concurrently for a more therapeutic effect.

Common Medications

Isoniazid (INH)
Paraminosalicylic acid (PAS)
Streptomycin (SM)
Ethambutol
Rifampin

Bronchodilators

Bronchodilators act by relaxing the smooth muscles of the bronchioles and are beneficial in controlling bronchospasm associated with chronic pulmonary diseases such as asthma, bronchitis, and emphysema. Most COPD patients are on some form of bronchodilator medication at home. Since most bronchodilators contain preparations of Aminophylline, epinephrine, or isoproterenol, it is important to relay to the base hospital information on any bronchodilator medications the patient is currently taking, as their current regimen may alter field treatment. Bronchodilators may be taken orally, by aerosol inhalers, and occasionally by suppository.

Common Medications

Aminophylline (theophylline)
Isuprel Mistometer
Metaprel (po or inhaler)
Tedral
Terbutaline
Bronkosol (IPPB)
Quibron
Marax
Bronkotabs

Cardiac Glycosides

Cardiac glycosides are digitalis preparations that are frequently prescribed for the management of chronic congestive heart failure and for the control of certain rhythm disturbances, specifically atrial fibrillation and atrial flutter. They act to improve myocardial contractility by increasing stroke volume and slowing the conduction through the SA and AV nodes. This improves cardiac output by allowing the ventricles to rest and fill more completely between contractions. Digitalis preparations also cause the heart to pump more efficiently and reduce myocardial oxygen consumption. Patients are commonly placed on digitalis preparations following myocardial infarction or acute episodes of congestive heart failure. When antiarrhythmic agents such as quinidine, Pronestyl, or Inderal are simultaneously prescribed, you should suspect that the patient had a previous myocardial infarction and anticipate arrhythmias.

Digitalis toxicity occurs occasionally in patients taking digitalis preparations and may be the reason you are called to the scene. Despite the frequent and early occurrences of gastrointestinal symptoms indicating digitalis toxicity, a disturbance of cardiac rhythm is usually the first evidence of toxicity. Frequently occurring arrhythmias include PVCs, first degree AV block, sinus arrest, SA block, atrial tachycardia with block, ventricular bigeminy, and even ventricular tachycardia. Other signs of toxicity include anorexia and visual disturbances such as diplopia, halo effect around dark objects, or a yellow or green tinge to objects.

Common Medications

Digoxin (Lanoxin)
Digitalis leaf
Digitoxin
Gitaligin

Diuretics

Patients are placed on oral diuretic agents at home to control the edema that frequently accompanies chronic congestive heart failure or renal insufficiency. Diuretics act by stimulating the kidneys to excrete excess water and sodium, usually by inhibiting the reabsorption of sodium at the renal tubules. Since potassium is excreted along with sodium and water, these patients are usually on concurrent potassium supplements. Excessive serum potassium depletion or elevation can induce ventricular arrhythmias.

Common Medications

Lasix
Diuril
Hydrodiuril (hydrochlorathiazide, HCTZ, Esidrex, Oretic)
Aldactone
Dyazide
Hygroton
Edecrin (ethacrinic acid)
Hydromox
Aldactazide
Naturetin
Aquatag (Edemex)
Anhydron
Saluron
Aquatensen
Naqua (Metahydrin)
Triamterene

Hormones

Hormones are complex chemical agents manufactured by the body's endocrine glands to control growth, sexual development, metabolism, and electrolyte balance. Occasionally a deficiency can occur which may require treatment by the administration of natural or synthetic hormones. Most oral contraceptives contain hormones. Hormone therapy has also been used to combat certain carcinomas.

Common Medications

Premarin
Provera, Depo–Provera
Diethylstilbestrol
Tace
Estradiol (Aquadiol, Delestrogen)
Estrone (Ogen, Femspan)
Synestrol
Hexadrol
Vallestril
Meprane
Amnestrogen (Evex, Menest)

Gesterol (progesterone, Lipo-Lutin, Proluton)
Nelalutin
Common Oral Contraceptives:
  Ovulen
  Demulen
  Norinyl
  Ortho-Novum
  Norlestrin
  Enovid
  Ovral
  Oracon
  Norquen

Hypoglycemic Agents

Hypoglycemic agents are used to control diabetes mellitus. This is a hereditary disease which results when the body is unable to metabolize glucose properly. These agents may be injected or taken orally, and the dosage varies according to the patient's health, diet, and exercise routine. Diabetics usually adjust their own medications, and occasionally they miscalculate, leading to hyper- or hypoglycemic states.

Common Medications

Insulins for injection:
  Regular (short-acting)
  NPH
  Lente
  Crystalline zinc
Oral hypoglycemics:
  Orinase
  Diabinese
  Talbutamide
  Dymelor
  Tolinase
  DBI

Laxatives and Stool Softeners

Laxatives and stool softeners are drugs that prevent constipation by generally altering fecal consistency and by stimulating peristalsis. They are dispensed in oral, liquid or suppository form and can be either prescribed or purchased "over the counter."

Most elderly or confined individuals are on some form of daily laxative, as inactivity contributes to constipation. Patients with gastrointestinal disorders may take these medications to control their condition.

Common Medications

Colace
Metamucil
Senakot
Ducolax
Milk of Magnesia (MOM)
Cascara
Castor oil
Mineral oil
Glycerin suppositories

Sedatives and Hypnotics

Sedatives are central nervous system depressants used to calm nervousness, irritability, and excitement. Hypnotics are agents which are used to induce sleep. Both groups of these drugs may be abused and can lead to respiratory depression, coma, and death.

Common Medications

Sedatives:
  Valium
  Librium
  Phenobarbital
  Thorazine
Hypnotics:
  Nembutal (pentobarbital)
  Seconal (secobarbital)
  Tuinal
  Phenobarbital
  Quaalude (methaqualone)
  Chloral hydrate
  Dalmane
  Placidyl
  Noludar
  Equanil (Miltown)

Steroids

Steroids are effective in treating chronic adrenocortical insufficiency, allergic reactions, collagen disorders, and other inflammatory processes. Although the method by which steroids control inflammatory processes is not fully understood, they have a wide spectrum of application. Patients on steroid therapy may experience mild GI bleeding and a diminished resistance to infection. If the patient is not being closely managed, he may suffer an adrenocortical crisis, especially when being weaned off steroids. A controlled, gradual weaning will allow the body to adjust to the decreased level of circulating steroids.

Common Medications

Prednisolone
Prednisone
Dexamethasone (Decadron, Hexadrol)
Cortisone acetate
Hydrocortisone
Solu–Cortef
Solu–Medrol
Florinef acetate

Sulfonamides

Sulfonamides are broad spectrum bacteriostatic drugs frequently used in the treatment of urinary tract infections. Like penicillin they may provoke an allergic reaction. Listed below are several sulfonamides and penicillins as well as other unrelated drugs commonly prescribed for the treatment of urinary tract infections.

Common Medications

Gantrisin (sulfasoxazole)
NegGram
Pyridium
Mandelamine
Furadantin
Bactrim
Septra
Gantanol
Sulfamylon acetate (mafenide acetate)
Macrodantin

SELF-ASSESSMENT QUESTIONS

AMINOPHYLLINE

1. Explain how Aminophylline works in an asthma patient. In a pulmonary edema patient.

2. What is the dose of Aminophylline and explain how it is administered?

3. What is the drug of choice in a child under 12 who is having an asthma attack?

4. What are the side effects of Aminophylline?

5. What arrhythmias are commonly seen with the administration of Aminophylline?

6. How can you determine the effectiveness of Aminophylline?

AMMONIA INHALANT

1. When is it appropriate to use ammonia ampules?

2. Explain the action of ammonia.

3. In which patients should ammonia be used with caution? Why?

4. Discuss the administration of Ammonia.

ARAMINE

1. How does Aramine increase blood pressure?

2. Give the dosage(s) and route(s) of Aramine.

3. Which arrhythmias may be caused by the administration of Aramine?

4. What side effects may occur if Aramine is administered too rapidly?

5. Why must the Aramine flow rate be increased *gradually*?

6. Discuss the field use of Aramine.

ATROPINE SULFATE

1. Since Atropine is a parasympathetic blocker, what are its effects on the heart?

2. When is Atropine indicated?

3. Explain why Atropine is not effective in a complete heart block with an underlying escape idioventicular rhythm.

4. What is the dosage and route of Atropine for heart blocks?

5. What is the dosage and route of Atropine for organophosphate poisoning?

6. What are the signs and symptoms of Atropine toxicity?

7. Why should Atropine be used with caution in glaucoma patients? In an MI patient?

8. How do you measure the effectiveness of Atropine in organophosphate poisoning?

9. Explain how Atropine works in organophosphate poisoning.

10. Can Atropine be used to treat PVCs in a bradycardia? Explain why or why not.

BENADRYL

1. Why is Benadryl used in anaphylaxis?

2. Give the dosage and routes of Benadryl.

3. Explain why Benadryl is contraindicated in the presence of alcohol or depressant drugs.

4. Why is Benadryl contraindicated in an asthma attack?

5. List two actions of Benadryl.

CALCIUM CHLORIDE

1. When is $CaCl_2$ indicated?

2. What are the side effects of $CaCl_2$?

3. Give the dose and routes of $CaCl_2$.

4. Why is $CaCl_2$ given in electromechanical dissociation?

5. Why should $CaCl_2$ be administered slowly when given IV push?

6. What complication can occur if $CaCl_2$ is administered with sodium bicarbonate?

DEXTROSE, 50%

1. When is 50% Dextrose indicated in the prehospital setting?

2. Give the usual dosage and routes of administration of 50% Destrose.

3. What complication can occur if 50% Dextrose infiltrates?

4. How can you assure that infiltration does not occur during injection of 50% Dextrose?

5. Why is 50% Dextrose not contraindicated in a suspected hyperglycemic patient?

6. What procedure should always preceed the administration of any glucose preparation and why?

EPINEPHRINE 1 : 10,000

1. Epinephrine 1 : 10,000 is utilized in the treatment of what conditions?

2. Discuss the pharmacologic action of Epinephrine on the:
   a. heart
   b. periphery

3. Give the usual dosage and route(s) of Epinephrine 1 : 10,000.

4. How would you determine the effectiveness of Epinephrine after administration?

5. How could you convert Epinephrine 1 : 10,000 to 1 : 10,000 for intravenous administration?

6. What are possible side effects of administering Epinephrine?

EPINEPHRINE 1 : 1,000

1. Epinephrine 1 : 1000 is used in the field treatment of what conditions?

2. What effect does Epinephrine have on the bronchi and the periphery?

3. Give the usual dosage and route of administration of Epinephrine 1 : 1000.

4. Why is this concentration of Epinephrine (1 : 1000) not given IV push?

5. What is the main side effect of Epinephrine?

6. How do you judge the effectiveness of Epinephrine?

7. Epinephrine should be used cautiously in treating patients with which conditions?

8. Why is Epinephrine sometimes given at the site of an insect sting? In which cases is this procedure contraindicated?

9. Why would a subcutaneous injection of Epinephrine 1 : 1000 be ineffective in the presence of circulatory collapse? What dosage and route of Epinephrine would then be indicated?

GLUCOLA

1. Discuss the actions of Glucola.

2. List some field uses of Glucola.

3. Give the usual dosage and route of administration for Glucola.

4. When would Glucola be contraindicated?

5. How would you assess the patient's ability to swallow Glucola without aspirating?

6. What procedure must be performed before administering Glucola?

7. How is Glucola ordered in the pediatric patient?

INDERAL

1. When should Inderal be indicated in the prehospital setting?

2. Discuss the actions of Inderal.

3. Give the dosage, route, and method of administration for Inderal.

4. When would Inderal be administered with caution?

5. What side effects can occur following Inderal administration?

6. How might you help prevent side effects of Inderal?

7. What procedures might you try before using Inderal?

8. Inderal is ordered in the oral form for the control of which two clinical conditions?

INSTANT GLUCOSE PASTE

1. When would you most likely use Instant Glucose Paste in the field?

2. Discuss the action of Instant Glucose Paste in a hypoglycemic patient.

3. Give the dosage, route and method of administration of Instant Glucose Paste.

4. How can you prevent aspiration in a comatose patient to whom you have given Instant Glucose Paste?

INTROPIN

1. Discuss the use of Intropin in the field management of shock.

2. List the actions of Intropin.

3. Discuss how Intropin increases blood pressure.

4. Discuss the dosage and route of administration of Intropin.

5. Give the major side effects that can occur with Intropin administration.

6. When is Intropin contraindicated?

7. What clinical signs and symptoms would you expect to find if you were infusing Intropin too rapidly?

8. What complication can occur if the Intropin drip infiltrates? What should then be done?

IPECAC
(Syrup of)

1. What would you do if a patient to whom you were going to give Ipecac suddenly became unreponsive?

2. What is the usual dosage of Ipecac for adults? For small children?

3. How does Ipecac work to induce vomiting?

4. Why is it important to dilute Ipecac with large amounts of clear fluid?

5. Ipecac is contraindicated in what types of ingested agents?

6. When is Ipecac indicated for field use?

ISUPREL

1. What are the actions of Isuprel?

2. Isuprel is the drug of choice to treat which arrhythmias?

3. What is the dosage range of Isuprel?

4. An Isuprel drip is titrated to which vital sign?

5. What are possible side effects of Isuprel administration?

6. With which drug does Isuprel have a cumulative effect?

ISUPREL MISTOMETER

1. How do you administer a dosage of Isuprel from an Isuprel Mistometer?

2. What is the action of Isuprel when administered via the Mistometer?

3. When might you use the Isuprel Mistometer?

4. What are the side effects to watch for when using the Isuprel Mistometer?

5. When is it contraindicated to use the Isuprel Mistometer, and why?

6. Patients who over-use their Isuprel Mistometer may develop what response?

LANOXIN

1. When would Lanoxin be indicated in the field situation?

2. How does Lanoxin work to modify the heart rate?

3. Give the usual dose and route for Lanoxin.

4. Discuss the contraindications of Lanoxin administration.

5. Describe the normal side effects of Lanoxin.

6. List the signs and symptoms of digitalis toxicity.

7. What arrhythmias usually present with digitalis toxicity?

LASIX

1. What is the dosage range for Lasix IV push in the field?

2. Lasix is used in the field treatment of what acute medical emergency?

3. What are the contraindications for the field use of Lasix?

4. What are the actions of Lasix?

5. Why is it important to report a patient's home use of oral diuretics to your base hospital?

LEVOPHED

1. What type of patients may require a Levophed drip?

2. What are two side effects of Levophed administration?

3. Give the dosage and route of administration for Levophed.

4. How does Levophed work to increase the blood pressure?

5. Which parameters must you monitor closely while administering Levophed?

6. What can happen if a Levophed drip infiltrates, and what should you do then?

7. Why might you need to use Atropine in conjunction with Levophed therapy?

MANNITOL

1. What are the actions of Mannitol?

2. What is the dosage range and route of administration for Mannitol?

3. List two possible side effects of Mannitol administration.

4. When is Mannitol contraindicated?

5. What must you watch for and monitor closely when administering Mannitol?

6. Discuss the effects of temperature changes on Mannitol.

7. What do you do if the Mannitol solution has crystalized in the bottle?

8. When would you use Mannitol in the field?

9. List the signs and symptoms of increased intracranial pressure.

MORPHINE SULFATE

1. List the actions of Morphine Sulfate.

2. What are the indications for field use of Morphine Sulfate?

3. What are the contraindications for field use of Morphine Sulfate?

4. How may Morphine Sulfate be administered and in what dosages?

5. What are the side effects of Morphine Sulfate administration?

6. Discuss the desired effects of Morphine Sulfate.

NARCAN

1. What are the routes for Narcan administration?

2. What is the adult dosage of Narcan? The pediatric dose?

3. List the drugs against which Narcan is effective.

4. List two uses for Narcan.

5. List the side effects and contraindications of Narcan.

6. Why would you delay inserting an esophageal obturator airway in a patient in whom you intend to administer Narcan?

7. Once a patient responds to Narcan, why is it important to monitor him closely?

NITROGLYCERIN

1. What are common names for Nitroglycerin?

2. How is Nitroglycerin administered?

3. What is the dosage of Nitroglycerin?

4. How does Nitroglycerin reduce myocardial oxygen consumption?

5. List the side effects of Nitroglycerin.

6. What are the contraindications of Nitroglycerin administration?

7. Discuss the importance of taste in evaluating the potency of Nitroglycerin.

8. Why does Nitroglycerin need to be replaced every six months?

PHYSOSTIGMINE

1. How does Physostigmine counteract the effects of tricyclic antidepressants and belladonna alkaloids?

2. Name specific tricyclic drugs which Physostigmine counteracts.

3. Discuss the dosage and route of administration for Physostigmine.

4. List the side effects associated with Physostigmine administration.

5. Discuss the contraindications for the use of Physostigmine.

6. What drug is an antagonist to Physostigmine?

7. What clinical parameters do you use to monitor the effectiveness of Physostigmine?

8. What can occur if Physostigmine is administered too rapidly?

PITOCIN

1. When is Pitocin used in the field?

2. Discuss the action of Pitocin.

3. What are possible side effects with the use of Pitocin?

4. Discuss the dosage(s) and route(s) of Pitocin administration.

5. Give two contraindications for the use of Pitocin.

6. Why is Pitocin *not* administered prior to the delivery of the infant and placenta?

7. List two nonpharmacological methods for controlling postpartum hemorrhage.

SODIUM BICARBONATE

1. How does Sodium Bicarbonate reduce acidosis?

2. What are the field indications for the use of Sodium Bicarbonate?

3. How is Sodium Bicarbonate administered, and what determines the dosage?

4. What condition results from over-administration of Sodium Bicarbonate?

5. What can occur with the administration of Sodium Bicarbonate in a well–ventilated patient?

6. What drug will precipitate when mixed with Sodium Bicarbonate?

VALIUM

1. How does Valium reduce seizure activity?

2. Why is Valium used before cardioverting?

3. In which seizure situations is Valium indicated?

4. What are the dosages and routes of administration of Valium?

5. What may occur if IV Valium is administered too rapidly; what action would you then take?

6. When will IV Valium precipitate and how can this be prevented?

XYLOCAINE

1. When would you use Xylocaine in the field?

2. What is the action of Xylocaine?

3. When is Xylocaine contraindicated?

4. How do you administer Xylocaine and why?

5. What are the early and late side effects of Xylocaine administration?

6. What would you do if a patient showed early signs of Xylocaine toxicity?

7. What is the maximum dosage of Xylocaine to be administered over one hour?

5% DEXTROSE IN WATER

1. How is D_5W most commonly used?

2. When is D_5W contraindicated?

NORMAL SALINE

1. When is normal saline most commonly used?

2. When is normal saline contraindicated?

3. How is the drip rate of normal saline determined?

RINGER'S LACTATE

1. When is Ringer's Lactate indicated over other IV solutions?

2. What precautions must be taken when administering Ringer's Lactate to a patient with a head injury?

3. List 3 medical conditions where Ringer's Lactate would be an appropriate IV solution to administer.

4. Why is a large bore cannula needle indicated with Ringer's Lactate?

SALT POOR ALBUMIN

1. How does Salt Poor Albumin expand blood volume?

2. List and explain the major contraindications for the use of Salt Poor Albumin.

3. What early physical findings might suggest adverse effects of Salt Poor Albumin?

4. Explain the dosage of Salt Poor Albumin.

5. In what conditions might Salt Poor Albumin be ordered in the field?

METRIC CONVERSION TABLES

Liquid Equivalents

Metric System	Apothecary System
1000 ml (1 liter)	1 quart (32 fl oz)
500 ml	1 pint (16 fl oz)
250 ml	1 cup (8 fl oz)
30 ml	1 fluid ounce
15 ml	1 Tablespoon (Tbs)
4–5 ml	1 teaspoon (fluid dram)
1 ml = 1 cc	15 minims

CONVERSIONS:

A. To convert cc to Tbs divide by 15 cc
   Example: 45 cc ÷ 15 cc/Tbs = 3 Tbs
B. To convert Tbs to cc multiply by 15 cc
   Example: 6 Tb × 15 cc/Tbs = 90 cc

METRIC CONVERSION TABLES

Weight Equivalents

Metric System	Apothecary System
1 kilogram (kg)	2.2 pounds (lb) 1 pound = 16 ounces (oz)
30 g	1 oz
1 g = 1000 mg	15 grains
60 mg	1 grain
1 mg	1/60 grain

CONVERSIONS:

A. To convert mg to grains divide by 60
   Example: 300 mg ÷ 60= 5 grains
B. To convert grains to mg multiply by 60
   Example: 0.25 grain × 60= 15 mg
C. To convert lb to kg divide by 2.2
   Example: 77 lb ÷ 2.2 = 35 kg
D. To convert kg to lb mulitply by 2.2
   Example: 40 kg × 2.2 = 88 lb
E. To convert mg to g divide by 1000
   Example: 6000 mg ÷ 1000 = 6 g
F. To convert g to mg multiply by 1000
   Example: 1 g × 1000 = 1000 mg

METRIC CONVERSION TABLES

Average Weight/Age for Pediatric Patients

Age	Weight (lb)	Weight (kg)
Birth	7	3.5
3 mo	10	5
6 mo	15	7
9 mo	18	8
1 yr	22	10
2 yr	26	12
3 yr	33	15
4 yr	37	17
5 yr	40	18
6 yr	44	20
7 yr	50	23
8 yr	56	25
9 yr	60	28
10 yr	70	33
11 yr	75	35
12 yr	85	40
13 yr	98	44

Calculation and Regulation of IV Drip Rates

Administration sets made by various manufacturers are constructed to yield varying numbers of drops per cubic centimeter. This information may be found on the box containing the set.

10 drops (gtt)/cc Travenol

Basic formula for calculating the regulation of IV fluids:

$$\frac{\text{Total volume infused} \times \text{gtt/cc}}{\text{Total time for infusion in minutes}} = \text{gtt/minute}$$

With pediatric (micro) administration sets, no conversion factor is needed.

Pediatric sets deliver 60 μgtt/cc,
therefore cc/hr = μgtt/minute

METRIC CONVERSION TABLES

Travenol IV Drip Rate

gtt/Min (10 gtt/ml)	Rate of Infusion ml/hr
5.0	30
	35
6.0	40
7.0	45
8.0	50
10.0	60
11.0	65
12.0	70
	75
13.0	80
15.0	90
17.0	100
20.0	120
21.0	125
23.0	140
25.0	150
33.0	200
42.0	250

Calculation of IV Medication Drip Rates

You have one gram of Lidocaine in 500 cc of D_5W. How many microdrips per minute do you need to deliver?

1 mg/min _____

2 mg/min _____

3 mg/min _____

4 mg/min _____

Step 1:   Convert grams to milligrams
$$1 \text{ gm} = 1000 \text{ mg}$$

Step 2:   Find the number of mg per cc of solution by dividing the amount of solution (in cc) into the amount of drug (in mg).

$$500 \text{ cc } \overline{\big) 1{,}000 \text{ mg}} = 2 \text{ mg/cc}$$

215

METRIC CONVERSION TABLES
Continued

Step 3:   Once you find the number of mg per cc of solution you can use the desired (D) over have (H) formula to determine the number of cc/min to be delivered.

$$\frac{D}{H} \quad \frac{1 \text{ mg/min}}{2 \text{ mg/cc}} = 0.5 \text{ cc/min}$$

Step 4:   Once you find the number of cc/min you wish to deliver, multiply this by the number of gtt/cc your infusion set delivers.
(Remember that 60 microdrips is always equal to one cc)

   0.5 cc/min × 60 gtt/cc = 30 gtt/min. Therefore, to deliver 1 mg/min you infuse 30 gtt/min.

METRIC CONVERSION
SELF-ASSESSMENT QUESTIONS
Medications

1. You are ordered to add 1.5 mg of Isuprel to 500 cc of D_5W. You have Isuprel 5 mg in a 5 cc vial. How many cc do you add?

2. An MD orders 30 cc of Ipecac to be given to an overdose patient. How many tablespoons do you give?

3. You have 15 mg of MS in a 1 cc vial. You are ordered to give gr ⅛ MS. IM. You administer how many ccs?

4. Lasix comes in 2 cc amps containing 20 mg. The physician orders 100 mg IV STAT. How many ccs do you give?

5. You are ordered to give 250 mg of Aminophylline IV slowly. You have 1 gm in 10 cc. How many ccs do you give?

6. For postpartum hemorrhage, you are asked to give Pitocin 4 Units in an IV drip. You find the vial labeled 10 Units per cc. How many ccs do you draw up in your syringe?

7. You are to give 500 mg of Calcium Chloride IV. You have 1 gm in 10 cc. How many ccs do you give?

8. You have 100 mg of lidocaine in a 10 cc preloaded syringe. You are ordered to give 75 mg. How many ccs do you give?

9. You have atropine vial which has 0.5 mg per cc. The MD wants you to give 1.0 mg IV bolus. What is the correct dose in ccs?

IV Fluid Drip Rates

1. You are ordered to start an IV of Ringer's Lactate. Using a standard drip (10 gtt/cc), how many gtt/min do you need to adjust your flow rate to achieve a rate of:
    a. 300 cc/hr:
    b. 180 cc/hr:
    c. 500 cc/hr:
    d. 250 cc/hr:

2. The Base Station orders Aminophylline 250 mg in 20 cc D_5W over 30 minutes via volutrole drip. You have available 250

METRIC CONVERSION
SELF-ASSESSMENT QUESTIONS

mg/10 cc. How fast should you run your microdrip rate to infuse the 30 cc contained in the volutrol?

3. You are ordered to start an IV of Ringer's Lactate in a trauma patient as a precautionary measure in case his vital signs deteriorate and volume replacement is required. Using the maxidrip, how many gtt/min equals the ordered rate of 30 cc/hr?

IV Medication Drip Rates

1. You are ordered to prepare a Lidocaine drip to control PVCs. Using a microdrip, calculate the number of gtt/min that would give you the following mg/min:
   a. 1 gm in 250 cc D_5W at 4 mg/min:
   b. 2 gm in 500 cc D_5W at 2 mg/min:
   c. 2 gm in 250 cc D_5W at 4 mg/min:

2. The formula for the *maximum* amount of Lidocaine that can be safely infused over one hour is *4 mg/kg/hr*. You have a 176 pound man and are ordered to mix Lidocaine 2 gm/500 cc D_5W:
   a. What is the maximum amount of Lidocaine he can receive over one hour?
   b. How many mg/cc are there in the mixture of Lidocaine 2 gm/500 cc D_5W?
   c. You have already given a 100 mg Lidocaine bolus. Subtracting that, how many more mg of Lidocaine can be safely administered over one hour?
   d. You are ordered to run your Lidocaine drip at 3 mg/min. Is this a safe rate or a rate exceeding the safe formula of 4 mg/kg/hr?

ANSWERS TO METRIC CONVERSION SELF-ASSESSMENT QUESTIONS

Medications
1. 1.5 cc
2. 2 Tbl
3. 0.5 cc
4. 10 cc
5. 2.5 cc
6. 0.4 cc
7. 5 cc
8. 7.5 cc
9. 2 cc

IV Fluid Drip Rates
1. a. 50 gtt/min
   b. 30 gtt/min
   c. 83 gtt/min
   d. 42 gtt/min
2. 60 gtt/min
3. 5 gtt/min

IV Medication Drip Rates
1. a. 60 gtt/min
   b. 30 gtt/min
   c. 30 gtt/min
2. a. 320 mg
   b. 4 mg/cc
   c. 220 mg
   d. safe rate

ARRHYTHMIAS

INTRODUCTION

This section is not designed to teach arrhythmias, but is merely intended to review the basic principles of electrocardiography and arrhythmia interpretation. It is not a substitute for a course in electrocardiography. Arrhythmia interpretation is often difficult and should only be approached if you have had actual training in interpreting EKGs, since inexperienced persons can easily become confused and develop misconceptions that are difficult to correct.

The EKG section has been organized to review arrhythmias in a systematic manner. First, there is a general review of electrophysiology and the principles of electrocardiography. Following this, each of the most common arrhythmias is discussed in order of its occurrence within the conduction system. Each narrative includes a summary of etiology, identifying EKG features, clinical picture, and treatment of these types of cardiac problems.

The discussion of common arrhythmias is followed by a brief description of several electrocardiographic phenomena which may confuse or modify your interpretation of arrhythmias. These include topics such as escape mechanism and bundle branch block.

Finally, there is a self-assessment section which includes questions on basic principles as well as a variety of patient situations which require arrhythmia interpretation and management. All of the EKG strips in this section should be interpreted as being Lead II.

In utilizing this section for review, avoid the temptation to use pattern recognition of the EKG strips. Instead, visualize and understand the physiologic activity within the heart that produced the arrythmia and the expected clinical manifestations. Use a consistent organized approach to gather all the information available from the EKG and compare it to the identifying features listed for each arrhythmia prior to your interpretation. The rates quoted for the various arrhythmias are to be used solely as guidelines for clinical interpretation of the EKG strip, and should not be considered inflexible standards.

All cardiac arrhythmias should be evaluated for their effect on cardiac output or their potential for progression to a lethal arrhythmia. Determine the required treatment by assessing the patient thoroughly, as well as identifying the arrhythmia.

Begin this section by reviewing all of the basic EKG principles, then answer the questions and approach the clinical situations. After you have completed the Self-Assessment section, turn to the answer key and compare it to your own interpretations and treatments. Concentrate on weak areas and seek additional help from your instructor, your base hospital personnel, and the reference texts listed at the end of this manual until you are comfortable in your knowledge of arrhythmias.

ELECTROPHYSIOLOGY

The heart is composed of two types of cells which enable it to perform two distinct functions:

Electrical: Specialized cells which make up the conduction system and have the specific ability to initiate and transmit electrical activity in the heart.

Mechanical: Myocardial cells which make up the bulk musculature of the heart and contract in response to electrical stimuli.

The electrical impulse is responsible for stimulating the heart's mechanical contraction and is necessary for the heart to pump effectively. Although arrhythmias affect mechanical activity, they are caused by malfunctions in the electrical system. Therefore, in order to understand arrhythmias it is vital to understand the normal conduction system and how it works. The physical layout of the heart's electrical conduction system is diagrammed in Figure 4.1.

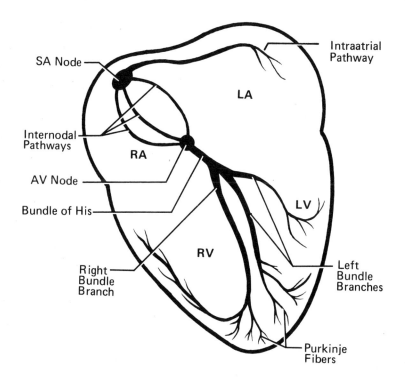

Figure 4.1. Electrical conduction system of the heart.

225

Electrical activity begins in the sinoatrial (SA) node and flows toward the ventricles. All areas of the conduction system have the ability to 1) initiate impulses, 2) become irritable, and 3) respond to an impulse.

Each area of the conduction system initiates impulses at its own inherent rate as shown here.

SA node	60–100/min
AV Junction	40–60/min
Ventricle	20–40/min

In general, the fastest pacemaker site will predominate and determine the heart rate.

The SA node is the usual pacemaker site since it initiates impulses at a faster rate than the junction or ventricle. However, if for some reason the SA node should fail, an impulse from the AV junction can "escape" and take over to pace the heart. Likewise, if the junction also fails, the ventricle can then take over. This protective backup system helps maintain the heart's electrical efficiency. There are times, however, when the junction or the ventricle becomes "irritable" and initiates impulses at a faster than normal rate, thus overriding the SA node and taking over control of the heart.

Innervation

Heart rate and myocardial contractility are influenced by the autonomic nervous system (ANS) via *sympathetic* and/or *parasympathetic stimulation*. Normal function is dependent on the proper balance of these two systems. However, if one or the other is either stimulated or blocked, the balance will be disrupted, resulting in abnormal function of the conduction system and subsequent arrhythmias. The ANS control of the heart is outlined in Figure 4.2.

Graphic Display of EKG

The electrical forces within the heart can be detected by electrodes attached to the patient's skin. If the flow of current is *toward* the positive electrode, the graphic display will depict a positive or upright mark on the EKG paper. If the flow is *away from* the positive electrode, the EKG deflection will be negative, or downward. Since the main flow of electrical activity in the heart travels from the SA node to the ventricles, the current is normally moving toward the positive electrode in Lead II. This produces a primarily upright

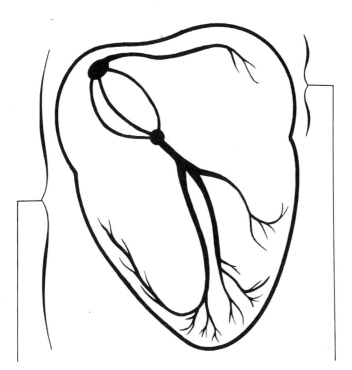

SYMPATHETIC

● Innervates both
  atria and ventricles

● Increases

  heart rate
  AV conduction
  irritability

PARASYMPATHETIC

● Innervates the atria
  via vagus nerve

● Little or no effect on
  junction or ventricles

● Decreases

  heart rate
  AV conduction
  irritability

Figure 4.2. Innervation of the heart.

complex with clearly visible P waves, which makes Lead II a valuable monitoring lead.

The basis for EKG interpretation is the use of a consistent medium for producing the written display of electrical activity. To serve this purpose, all EKG graph paper is uniform in its markings and the speed of the EKG machine or oscilloscope is standardized. By matching the markings made by the patient's electrical activity to the time and voltage measures on the graph paper, you can calculate the measurements of the patient's complex and compare them to "normal" or the preillness state. Standard measurements are shown in Figure 4.3.

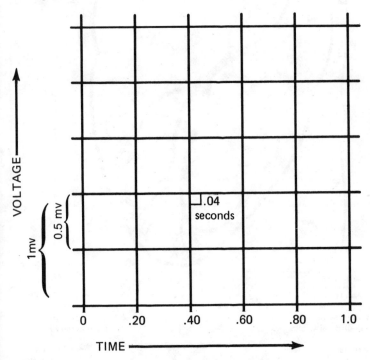

Figure 4.3. Standard graph paper measurements.

During each phase of the cardiac cycle, the electrical activity within the heart produces a distinct wave pattern on the graph paper. (Fig. 4.4)

Each of the features of the EKG cycle is uniformly defined (Fig. 4.5) regardless of the underlying rhythm.

If possible, the myocardial cells will respond to each electrical stimulus by contracting, thus producing a pulse. The electrical impulses that stimulate the heart beat are displayed in Figure 4.6.

Electrical Activity	Associated Pattern	Graphic Depiction
Atrial Depolarization	P Wave	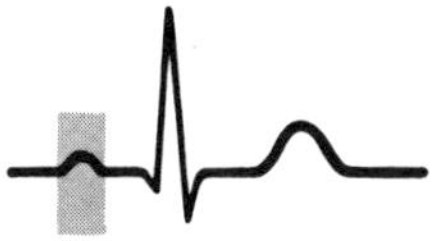
Delay at AV Node	PR Segment	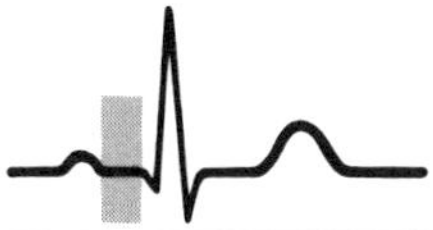
Ventricular Depolarization	QRS Complex	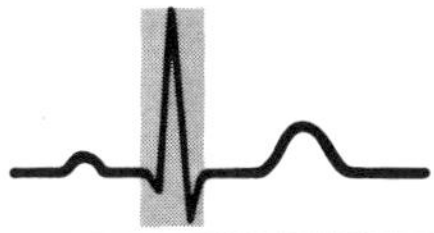
Ventricular Repolarization	T Wave	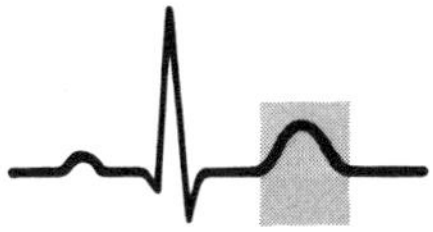
No electrical activity	Isoelectric Line	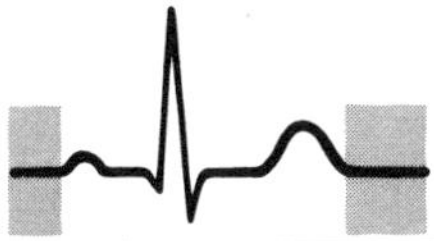

Figure 4.4. EKG wave patterns produced by electrical activity in the heart.

Electrical Refractoriness

When the heart is responding actively to an electrical stimulus, it cannot accept another stimulus and is totally unresponsive or "refractory". This phase of the cardiac cycle is called the *absolute* refractory period (ARP) and is diagrammed in Figure 4.7.

Refractoriness is a protective mechanism that prevents the heart from responding to all of the impulses fired by an excessively rapid pacemaker. At the end of the repolarization phase, some of the cells

EKG Display

EKG Component	Definition	Graphic Depiction
PR Segment	from the end of the P wave to the beginning of the QRS complex	
PRI	from the beginning of the P wave to the beginning of the QRS complex (normally .12-.20 seconds)	
Q Wave	first negative deflection of the QRS complex	
R Wave	first positive deflection of the QRS complex	
S Wave	first negative deflection following the R wave	
QRS Complex	from the beginning of the Q wave to the end of the S wave (normally less than .12 seconds)	
ST Segment	from the end of the S wave to the beginning of the T wave	

Figure 4.5. EKG wave, segment and internal definitions.

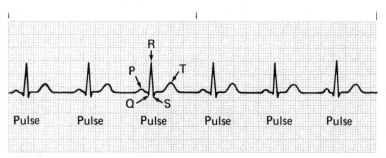

Figure 4.6. Display of electrical impulses on EKG paper. When assessing pulses, they should correspond to R waves.

230

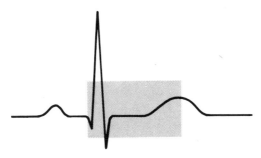

Figure 4.7. Absolute refractory period.

will recover before others and will be able to accept a new impulse if it is strong enough. This phase is called the *relative* refractory period (RRP) (Fig. 4.8).

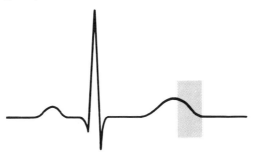

Figure 4.8. Relative refractory period.

If a strong stimulus falls during the relative refractory period, it may depolarize some of the cells while others remain refractory. This "sloppy" discharge can cause sudden ventricular irritability including arrhythmias such as ventricular tachycardia or ventricular fibrillation. Therefore, the relative refractory period is called the vulnerable phase of the cardiac cycle and becomes important if ventricular ectopics begin to occur on or near the T wave.

Approach to Arrhythmias

When analyzing an arrhythmia, you must be able to identify the electrical activity within the heart that produced the pattern. It isn't as important to be able to name the rhythm as it is to understand its mechanism and its effect on the patient. For this reason, it is vitally important that you avoid the temptation to use pattern recognition of arrhythmias. Instead, develop a consistent method for approaching rhythm strips and employ it with every arrhythmia you interpret. You will soon find yourself using it automatically, and only thinking of it consciously when you come to a difficult arrhythmia.

When analyzing an arrhythmia, ask yourself what's happening within that heart. Locate each of the P waves, then the QRS complexes. Next evaluate the relationship between them as shown by the PR intervals (PRIs). This should explain the interrelation of atrial activity to ventricular activity. The rate and rhythm will give you some idea of the effectiveness of the pattern and the impact it will have on the patient's cardiac output. When it comes time to treat, it is the patient who receives the drug, not the EKG strip, so look at your patient and assess perfusion. An example of an organized approach to arrhythmia interpretation is shown in Table 4.1.

Calculating Rates

There are several methods by which you can calculate the heart rate from an EKG tracing. All are based on the fact that vertical lines on the EKG paper are spaced .04 seconds apart. By measuring the R-R interval you can calculate the ventricular rate, while the P-P interval will measure the atrial rate. Both rates should be calculated on each rhythm strip to identify the relation between atrial and ventricular activity. Three rate calculation methods are shown in Table 4.2.

Table 4.1   Systematic Approach to Arrhythmia Interpretation

	Questions to ask	Things to consider
Rhythm:	Is it regular? Is it irregular? Are there any early beats? Are there any late beats?	If the R-R interval varies less than .04–.08 sec, it can be considered regular.
Rate:	What is the exact rate? Is it normal? Is it rapid? Is it slow? Is the atrial rate the	Rates are merely guidelines. Rates will frequently affect cardiac output and cause symptoms.

**Table 4.1 Systematic Approach to Arrhythmia
Interpretation (Continued)**

	Questions to ask	Things to consider
	same as the ventricular rate?	
P wave:	Is it present or not? Is the shape normal? Is it upright in Lead II? Is there one P for every QRS? Is the P in front of the QRS or behind it? Are there more Ps than QRSs? Do all the Ps look alike? Where are the dissimilar P waves?	The P wave is often the key to diagnosing the arrhythmia. If it's normal, the arrhythmia is of sinus origin. If it's flattened or otherwise unusual, it's atrial. If it's inverted, it's junctional. If it's absent, it could be atrial, junctional, or ventricular.
PR interval:	What is the PRI? Is it normal? Is it prolonged? Are all the PRIs constant? If the PRI is not constant is it getting longer?	If it's constant, there is conduction through the AV node If it varies, there is an AV disturbance. If it's longer than normal, there is delay in the AV node If there is no relation, they are dissociated
QRS complex:	What is the QRS? Is it of normal duration? Is it wider than normal? Do they all look alike? Does it have a normal relationship to the P?	If it's narrow, the arrhythmia is supraventricular. If it's wider than .12 it's probably ventricular; sometimes supraventricular arrhythmias have a wide QRS.

Table 4.2. Calculating Heart Rates

Method	Features
1500 divided by the number of small squares between 2 R waves	• most accurate • only used with regular rhythms • takes time to figure
No. of R waves in 6 sec. x 10	• very inaccurate • only good for irregular ryhthms • very quick estimate
300 divided by the number of large squares between 2 R waves **or**	• very quick • not very accurate with fast rates • only used with regular rhythms

Memorize This Scale

1 large square	= 300 beats/min
2 ” ”	= 150 beats/min
3 ” ”	= 100 beats/min
4 ” ”	= 75 beats/min
5 ” ”	= 60 beats/min
6 ” ”	= 50 beats/min

COMMON ARRHYTHMIAS

NORMAL SINUS RHYTHM

Etiology

Normal sinus rhythm (NSR) refers to the normal electrical pattern of the heart. In this rhythm, the SA node is the pacemaker and initiates electrical impulses which follow normal pathways and travel within normal time frames.

Identifying Features

Rhythm	regular
Rate	60–100 beats/min
P wave	normal and upright in Lead II
PR interval	.12–.20 seconds and constant
QRS	less than .12 seconds

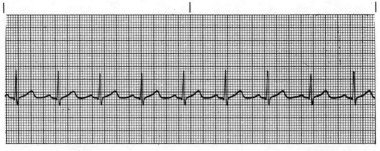

Normal Sinus Rhythm

Clinical Picture

Does not produce symptoms.

Treatment

Does not require treatment.

SINUS TACHYCARDIA

Etiology

In sinus tachycardia, the SA node is the pacemaker and discharges impulses at a rate greater than 100 beats/minute.

Conduction through the atria and ventricles is normal. The increased rate can be attributed to overactivity of the sympathetic nervous system or blocking of the parasympathetic nervous system. This may be caused by fever, anxiety, pain, or physical activity. Sinus tachycardia may also be an attempt to compensate for a drop in cardiac output.

Identifying Features

Rhythm	regular
Rate	greater than 100, usually 100–160 beats/min
P wave	normal and upright in Lead II
PR interval	.12–.20 seconds and constant
QRS	less than .12 seconds

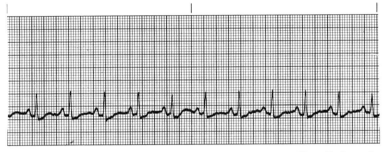

Sinus Tachycardia

Clinical Picture

- rapid regular pulse
- patient may complain of palpitations or dyspnea, or may be asymptomatic
- in the presence of an MI, may extend the infarction or induce CHF due to the increase in myocardial workload and oxygen consumption

Treatment

To treat this arrhythmia correctly you must identify the underlying cause by thorough history and physical exam and treat accordingly. It is not sufficient to merely slow the heart rate by vagotonic maneuvers and medications.

SINUS BRADYCARDIA

Etiology

In sinus bradycardia, the SA node is the pacemaker and discharges impulses at a rate of less than 60 beats/minute. Conduction follows the normal pathways. This slow rate is usually caused by increased parasympathetic (vagal) influence on the SA node. Other possible causes for a bradycardia include SA node damage, hypoxia, and drug overdose. Athletes frequently develop this rhythm as a result of prolonged physical exercise.

Identifying Features

Rhythm	regular
Rate	less than 60 beats/min
P wave	normal and upright in Lead II
PR interval	.12–.20 seconds and constant
QRS	less than .12 seconds

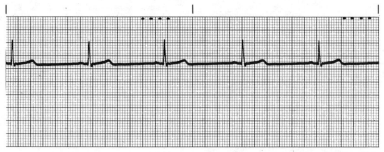

Sinus Bradycardia

Clinical Picture

- slow, regular pulse
- does not usually produce signs or symptoms of decreased cardiac output
- if rate is markedly slow, the decreased blood flow can lead to syncope or angina
- can be a warning of potential dangers such as blocks or asystole
- the slow rate can precipitate escape rhythms or ventricular irritability

Treatment

If the patient develops signs or symptoms of decreased cardiac output or ventricular irritability, treat the rhythm by increasing the heart rate. This usually may be accomplished with Atropine. Remember, PVCs associated with a bradycardia are *not* treated with Lidocaine.

SINUS ARRHYTHMIA

Etiology

In sinus arrhythmia, the SA node continues to be the pacemaker but discharges impulses at irregular intervals. This irregularity is caused by fluctuations in vagal activity during respiration. Heart rate increases with each inspiration and decreases with each expiration. This arrhythmia is very common in children.

Identifying Features

Rhythm	irregular
Rate	usually 60–100 beats/min
P wave	normal and upright in Lead II
PR interval	.12–.20 seconds and constant
QRS	less than .12 seconds

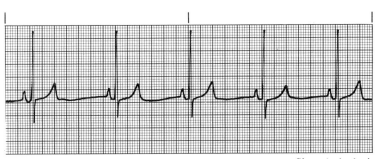

Sinus Arrhythmia

Clinical Picture

- irregular pulse

239

Treatment

Does not require treatment.

SA BLOCK OR SA ARREST

Etiology

In SA arrest the SA node fails to initiate an impulse at the expected time in the cardiac cycle. As a result an entire PQRST complex is absent because no other pacemaker site takes over pacing. In other instances the impulse is initiated normally but is blocked within the SA node and fails to reach the atria. Once again the entire PQRST complex is absent and this is called SA block. These arrhythmias may be caused by damage to the SA node, increased vagal influence, hypoxia, or drug overdose (especially Digoxin or Quinidine). If either of these arrhythmias persists, an escape beat may come in.

Identifying Features

Rhythm   normal except for missing beats
Rate   usually normal but frequently in the bradycardia range

P wave ⎫
PR interval ⎬ one or more entire PQRST complex(es) missing
QRS ⎭

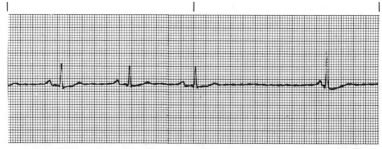

SA Block

Clinical Picture

- patient is usually unaware of this arrhythmia but may complain of feeling a skipped beat

- pulse will have a prolonged pause
- may develop signs or symptoms of cerebral ischemia if missed beats occur frequently

Treatment

SA arrest and SA block are usually self-limiting and the patient does not require treatment. Occasionally, frequent or prolonged periods of SA arrest or SA block may produce signs or symptoms of decreased cardiac output. If this occurs, atropine may be used to inhibit the vagal effect.

PREMATURE ATRIAL CONTRACTIONS

Etiology

A premature atrial contraction (PAC) occurs when an irritable focus in the atrium initiates an impulse which temporarily overrides the SA node. These premature beats can be distinguished from normal sinus beats because they occur early in the cardiac cycle and have a P wave of different morphology than the sinus beats, i.e., peaked, flattened, notched, diphasic or hidden in the T wave. PACs usually have normal conduction through the AV node and the ventricles. Atrial irritability is often indicative of myocardial damage, hypoxia, or drug overdose.

Identifying Features

Rhythm	regular, except for early beat
Rate	usually normal, depends on underlying arrhythmia
P wave	P wave of early beat differs from sinus beat, or may be lost in T wave
PR interval	.12–.20 seconds (may be prolonged) due to AV node refractoriness)
QRS	less than .12 seconds

241

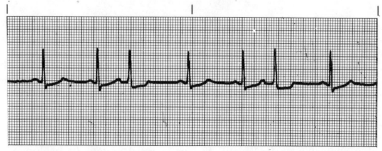

SR with PAC

Clinical Picture

- irregular pulse
- patient is unaware of premature beats but they may be detected by palpating a pulse or auscultating the heart
- positive identification can be made only by EKG

Treatment

Isolated PACs are of minimal significance and very often are corrected by oxygen alone. However, frequent PACs may be an early indication of CHF and may lead to atrial tachyarrhythmias. Therefore, watch the patient closely and treat the underlying cause of the PACs if indicated.

Special Note

Occasionally, a premature atrial beat will occur that is not conducted through the ventricles because they are refractory. This is called a nonconducted, or blocked, PAC. The P wave has different morphology than the sinus P wave, occurs early in the cardiac cycle and is not followed by a QRS complex. This arrhythmia is often confused with Mobitz II but can be differentiated by measuring the P-P interval. In Mobitz II, the P-P interval is regular, whereas a rhythm with a blocked PAC will produce an irregular P-P interval. If these beats occur frequently they can cause a drop in cardiac output.

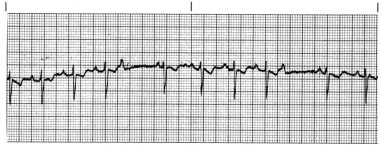

SR with Nonconducted PAC

ATRIAL TACHYCARDIA

Etiology

In atrial tachycardia, an irritable focus within the atrium suppresses activity of the SA node by initiating impulses at a rate of 150–250 beats/minute. Each impulse is conducted to the ventricles. The *atrial* P waves appear to be identical, but they do vary in morphology from the *sinus* P wave because they arise from a different focus. They may be peaked, flattened, notched, diphasic, or hidden in the T wave. If the P waves cannot be identified and ventricular conduction is normal, the arrhythmia is then described as a supraventricular tachycardia because it cannot be distinguished from a junctional tachycardia. Atrial tachycardia may be caused by myocardial damage, hypoxia, increased sympathetic influence or drugs.

Identifying Features

Rhythm   regular
Rate   150–250 beats/min
P wave   differs from sinus P wave, or may
            be lost in T wave
PR interval .12–.20 seconds
QRS   less than .12 seconds

243

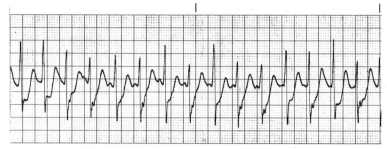

Atrial Tachycardia

Clinical Features

- rapid regular pulse
- patient is aware of increased heart rate and may exhibit signs or symptoms of decreased cardiac output or CHF
- atrial tachycardia is extremely dangerous in the presence of an MI because it increases myocardial oxygen consumption and workload

Treatment

This arrhythmia is usually converted by vagal stimulation such as Valsalva's maneuver or CSM. If these maneuvers are unsuccessful, medications such as digitalis or Inderal may be useful in slowing ventricular response or converting the arrhythmia. In extreme cases, when the patient's cardiac output has dropped and the above methods of conversion have failed, synchronized cardioversion may become necessary.

Special Note

When atrial tachycardia is paroxysmal in nature, that is, it starts and stops very suddenly, it is called Paroxysmal Atrial Tachycardia (PAT). Treatment is usually unnecessary because it doesn't last long and converts spontaneously.

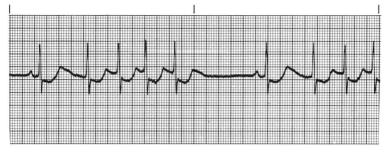

Paroxysmal Atrial Tachycardia

ATRIAL TACHYCARDIA WITH BLOCK

Etiology

When an atrial tachycardia (AT) has blocked ventricular conduction, it is called AT with block. The atrial rate is in the 150–250 range, thus differentiating it from atrial flutter. Conduction through ventricles is normal. Atrial tachycardia with block is usually indicative of organic heart disease but may also be caused by digitalis toxicity.

Identifying Features

Rhythm	regular, can be irregular if block is variable
Rate	*atrial rate,* 150–250 beats/min; *ventricular rate,* slower than atrial rate (depends on ratio of block)
P wave	atrial P wave, can look sawtoothed
PR interval	difficult to measure; normal
QRS	usually normal

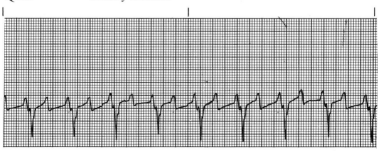

Atrial Tachycardia with Block

245

Clinical Picture

- will probably not produce signs or symptoms unless block is profound
- patient might be digitalis-toxic

Treatment

- Treatment is supportive. Check for digitalis toxicity.

ATRIAL FLUTTER

Etiology

Atrial flutter is caused by an irritable focus within the atrium which initiates regular impulses at a rate of 250–350 beats/minute, thus causing the atria to contract at an extremely rapid rate. To prevent all of the impulses from reaching the ventricles, the AV node blocks some of them, thereby creating a ratio between P waves and QRS complexes, usually in a pattern of 2:1, 4:1, or 6:1. Sometimes this conduction ratio varies, causing the ventricular rhythm to be irregular. Atrial conduction is represented by a sawtooth appearance and ventricular conduction is normal.

Identifying Features

Rhythm	atrial rhythm is regular; ventricular rhythm is usually regular but can be irregular if there is variable block
Rate	atrial rate 250–350 beats/min; ventricular rate varies
P wave	called "flutter waves," characteristic sawtooth pattern
PR interval	unable to measure
QRS	less than .12 seconds

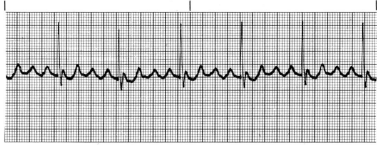

Atrial Flutter

Clinical Features

- can only be identified by EKG
- a rapid ventricular rate may cause the patient to complain of palpitations, angina, or dyspnea.
- a rapid ventricular rate and loss of the atrial kick can cause decreased cardiac output or increased myocardial oxygen consumption, which may in turn cause CHF or myocardial ischemia

Treatment

Field treatment is necessary only if the patient has a fast ventricular rate with signs or symptoms of decreased cardiac output. Treatment is aimed at terminating the atrial flutter or slowing the ventricular rate by increasing the block at the AV node. Field management includes Inderal, rapid–acting digitalis preparations, and/or cardioversion. Carotid sinus massage or other vagotonic maneuvers may be tried, but usually slow the rate temporarily rather than converting the arrhythmia.

ATRIAL FIBRILLATION

Etiology

In atrial fibrillation, the atria become extremely irritable, and many ectopic foci initiate impulses at a very rapid rate. Because the atria are bombarded by multiple impulses, they are unable to contract and merely quiver ineffectively. Since the atria are twitching, the atrial pattern on the EKG shows fibrillatory waves but no discernible P waves. Due to the inability of the ventricles to accept these rapid–fire stimuli, most of the atrial impulses are blocked at the AV node. Those impulses that are conducted reach the ventricles randomly, thus producing a grossly irregular ventricular rhythm. However, when atrial fibrillation becomes extremely rapid or extremely slow, it may have more regularity than usual. Atrial fibrillation is easily distinguished from other arrhythmias because it is *grossly irregular* and has *no discernible P waves.*

Identifying Features

Rhythm	grossly irregular
Rate	atrial rate greater than 400 beats/min
	ventricular rate varies greatly
P wave	no discernible P waves, atrial activity
	is referred to as fibrillatory waves
PR interval	unable to measure
QRS	less than .12 seconds

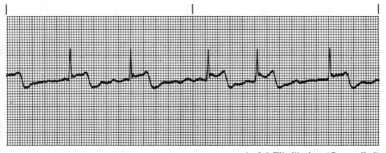

Atrial Fibrillation (Controlled)

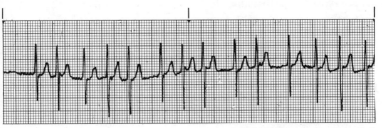

Atrial Fibrillation (Uncontrolled)

Clinical Picture

- irregular pulse
- patient may be aware of irregular heart beat and may complain of palpitations if ventricular rate is rapid

- may create a pulse deficit because the volume of blood ejected with every heart beat is not sufficient to produce a peripheral pulse
- may cause dyspnea or angina if the ventricular rate is rapid
- a rapid ventricular rate and the loss of the atrial kick can cause decreased cardiac output or increased myocardial oxygen consumption which may in turn cause CHF or myocardial ischemia
- patients have a tendency to develop thrombi in the non-contracting atrial chambers, with subsequent threat of embolization

Treatment

This can be a chronic rhythm. Many older patients encountered in the field will be in atrial fibrillation and not require treatment. However, if the patient is showing signs or symptoms of decreased cardiac output due to a rapid ventricular rate, treatment should be instituted at once. As with atrial flutter, CSM and other vagotonic maneuvers are usually unsuccessful, necessitating the use of a fast-acting digitalis preparation, Inderal, or even cardioversion.

WANDERING ATRIAL PACEMAKER

Etiology

The SA node is the primary pacemaker in wandering atrial pacemaker (WAP), but the site of impulse formation switches occasionally to the atrium or the junction. This may be caused by a speeding up of atrial or junctional impulses or by a slowing in the SA node due to sympathetic or parasympathetic influences. The shifting of pacemaker sites accounts for the variable P wave configuration. When the pacemaker site wanders toward or into the junction, the PRI may shorten or disappear. Conduction through the ventricles is normal.

Identifying Features

Rhythm	normal or slightly irregular
Rate	usually 60–100 beats/min

P wave	morphology changes
PR interval	less than .20 seconds; may vary
QRS	less than .12 seconds

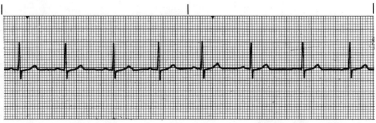

Wandering Atrial Pacemaker

Clinical Picture

- does not cause symptoms
- only identified by EKG

Treatment

No specific treatment for WAP. Watch for increasing incidence of junctional arrhythmias, as this may indicate myocardial irritability.

PREMATURE JUNCTIONAL CONTRACTION

Etiology

A premature junctional contraction (PJC) occurs when an irritable focus in the AV junction fires early and overrides the SA node. These ectopic beats can be distinguished from the sinus beats in Lead II because the P waves are inverted before or following the QRS complex, or are hidden in the QRS. The PRI is usually shortened and conduction through the ventricles is normal. An irritable junction may be caused by myocardial damage, hypoxia, or drugs.

Identifying Features

Rhythm	underlying rhythm is interrupted by the early beat

Rate	depends upon underlying rhythm
P wave	inverted before or after QRS, or hidden in QRS
PR interval	if P wave precedes QRS, PRI is usually .12 seconds or less
QRS	less than .12 seconds

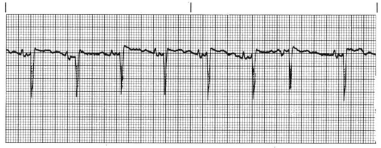

Sinus Rhythm with PJC

Clinical Features

- irregular pulse
- patients are usually unaware of premature beats because they rarely produce symptoms
- EKG is the only way to positively identify this arrhythmia

Treatment

Isolated PJCs are of little significance and can very often be alleviated by oxygen alone. Watch the patient closely for an increasing number of PJCs or the onset of junctional arrhythmias, as this may be indicative of increasing myocardial damage and irritability. If this occurs, you may use a Lidocaine drip, however this treatment is usually unsuccessful.

JUNCTIONAL RHYTHM

Etiology

If the SA node becomes damaged or receives increased vagal stimulation, it may lose its pacemaker role. When the SA node slows, an impulse from the junction may then assume control and become the pacemaker of the heart. This is a protective mechanism whereby the heart is able to continue to function despite failure of the SA node.

Impulses may originate in the upper, middle, or lower part of the AV junction, thereby causing various placement of the P wave in relation to the QRS complex. At the same time the impulse is being sent through the ventricles, it also travels retrograde through the atria causing an inverted P wave in Lead II. In rhythms originating in the upper junction, the P waves are inverted before the QRS complex, while the lower junction places the P wave after the QRS. If a PRI is present, it is shortened. If the impulse originates in the midjunction, both atria and ventricles will depolarize simultaneously and the P wave will be hidden in the QRS. Conduction through the ventricles is normal.

Identifying Features

Rhythm	regular
Rate	40–60 beats/min
P wave	inverted before or after the QRS, or hidden in QRS
PR interval	if P wave precedes QRS, PRI is usually .12 seconds or less
QRS	less than .12 seconds

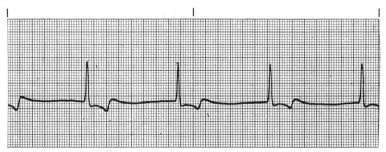

Junctional Rhythm

Clinical Features

- slow, regular pulse
- seldom produces signs or symptoms of decreased cardiac output
- can only be diagnosed by EKG

- may lead to heart blocks or ventricular standstill
- decreased cardiac output may occur and cause myocardial insufficiency
- may be an early sign of myocardial damage

Treatment

This rhythm is not usually treated, but if signs or symptoms of decreased cardiac output occur due to the slow ventricular rate, atropine, or possibly Isuprel may be necessary.

JUNCTIONAL TACHYCARDIA

Etiology

In junctional tachycardia, an irritable focus in the AV junction speeds up and overrides the SA node, thus becoming the pacemaker of the heart. Junctional tachycardia is an irritable arrhythmia, whereas a junctional escape rhythm is protective. Atrial activity is represented by inverted P waves before or following the QRS complex, or hidden in the QRS complex. The PRI is usually shortened, but conduction through the ventricles is normal. Damage to the AV junction is the usual cause of this arrhythmia but drug overdose such as digitalis toxicity may also be responsible.

This arrhythmia is often subdivided by rate as either accelerated junctional rhythm (60–100 beats/min) or junctional tachycardia (100–180 beats/min). Occasionally, junctional tachycardia will exceed a rate of 180 beats/min, but it is then very difficult to distinguish from AT, because P waves aren't visible, it is then termed supraventricular tachycardia.

Identifying Features

Rhythm	characteristically regular
Rate	60–180 (ocasionally exceeds 180) beats/min

Junctional Tachycardia

- 60–100 beats/min may be called accelerated junctional rhythm
- 100–180 beats/min may be called junctional tachycardia
- over 180 beats/min may be called supraventricular tachycardia

P wave	inverted before or after the QRS, or hidden in QRS
PR interval	if P wave precedes QRS, the PRI is usually .12 seconds or less
QRS	less than .12 seconds

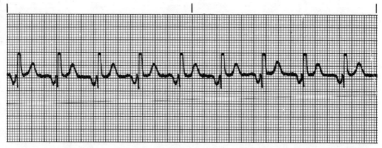

Accelerated Junctional Rhythm

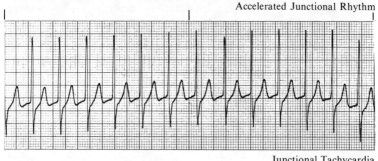

Junctional Tachycardia

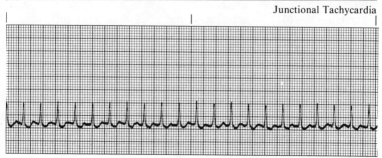

Supraventricular Tachycardia

Clinical Features

- if the rate is fast enough it may produce palpitations or symptoms of decreased cardiac output
- can only be diagnosed by EKG
- may progress to ventricular tachycardia or ventricular fibrillation
- usually indicative of advanced myocardial irritability

Treatment

If this arrhythmia is producing signs or symptoms of decreased cardiac output, the irritable focus must be suppressed immediately. Junctional tachycardia is usually converted by vagal stimulation such as Valsalva's maneuver or CSM. If these maneuvers are unsuccessful, medications such as digitalis or Inderal may be useful in slowing ventricular response or converting the arrhythmia. In extreme cases, when the patient's cardiac output has dropped and the above methods of conversion have failed, synchronized cardioversion may become necessary.

FIRST DEGREE AV BLOCK

Etiology

In the normal heart, impulses that arise in the SA node are delayed .12–.20 seconds at the AV node. In first degree heart block, this delay is prolonged resulting in a PRI that is longer than normal but constant. All impulses are then transmitted to the ventricle following normal ventricular conduction pathways. This arrhythmia may arise as a result of damage to the AV node, hypoxia, or drug overdose. You cannot completely identify an arrhythmia by calling it first degree heart block alone. To be complete, the underlying rhythm must also be identified.

Identifying Features

Rhythm	usually regular, depends on underlying rhythm
Rate	depends on underlying rhythm

P wave	normal and upright in Lead II, one P for each QRS
PR interval	greater than .20 seconds and constant
QRS	less than .12 seconds

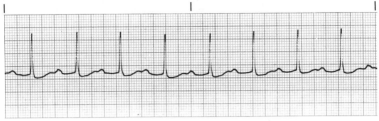

SR with 1st-degree AV Block

Clinical Picture

- patient is unaware of this arrhythmia
- no associated signs or symptoms
- can only be diagnosed by EKG
- not dangerous in itself but may forewarn of AV node injury which could lead to more advanced heart blocks
- a patient who has had a syncopal episode and is now in first degree heart block should be watched carefully for further block because he may be having Stokes-Adams attacks (transient syncopal episodes associated with intermittent periods of first and third degree heart block)

Treatment

First-degree heart block in itself does not require field treatment, but an underlying arrhythmia may require treatment if it is causing symptoms. Monitor the patient and transport to the hospital for follow-up care. Watch closely for increasing heart block especially in the presence of digitalis toxicity, myocardial infarction, or recent syncopal episodes.

SECOND DEGREE AV BLOCK
MOBITZ I (WENCKEBACH)

Etiology

In Wenckebach, the SA node continues to initiate impulses in a normal fashion, but the AV node becomes fatigued and fails to conduct the impulses to the ventricles in a reliable manner. The delay of each impulse at the AV node increases progressively until one is blocked completely. This causes the PRI to progressively lengthen until one QRS is "dropped." Once the beat is dropped, the cycle may repeat itself in a regular pattern. This pattern is often referred to as "grouped beating." Ventricular conduction remains normal. Wenckebach may be caused by damage to the AV node, hypoxia or drug overdose. It commonly occurs following an inferior MI and is considered relatively benign because the rate is usually adequate to maintain perfusion. However, it may progress to further heart block so monitor patient closely.

Identifying Features

Rhythm	atrial rhythm is regular; ventricular rhythm is irregular; R–R interval may become progressively shortened
Rate	atrial rate is normal; ventricular rate usually normal, can be slow and has intermittent dropped beats
P wave	normal and upright in Lead II; not every P wave has a QRS
PR interval	normal or greater than .20 seconds, becomes progressively longer until a P wave is not conducted, resulting in a dropped QRS
QRS	less than .12 seconds

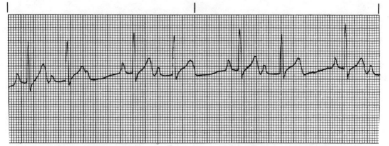

Mobitz I

Clinical Picture

- patient may notice irregularity of pulse
- can only be diagnosed by EKG
- a sudden drop in rate may cause signs or symptoms of decreased cardiac output

Treatment

Usually does not require field treatment. Occasionally, the rate may drop and cause signs or symptoms of decreased cardiac output, at which point atropine can be very effective in increasing the heart rate. Watch for the possibility of further heart block.

SECOND DEGREE AV BLOCK MOBITZ II (CLASSICAL)

Etiology

In Mobitz II, the SA node is the pacemaker and every beat is conducted normally to the AV node. Once reaching the AV node, however, only every second, third or fourth impulse is conducted through to the ventricles. Thus there is only one QRS complex for every two, three or four P waves. On the impulses that are conducted, the PRI may be normal or prolonged but it is *constant* with each conducted beat. The constant PRI is the key to diagnosing a Mobitz II. Conduction through the ventricles is normal. This arrhythmia may be caused by damage to the AV node, hypoxia, or drug overdose. Mobitz II is a dangerous arrhythmia because it may suddenly progress to third degree heart block or ventricular standstill.

258

Identifying Features

Rhythm	P to P interval is regular; R to R interval is usually regular but can be irregular
Rate	atrial rate is usually normal; ventricular rate is usually 1/2 to 1/3 that of the atrial rate
P waves	normal and upright in Lead II, more than one P wave for every QRS
PR interval	may be normal or prolonged, but is *constant* on conducted beats
QRS	less than .12 seconds

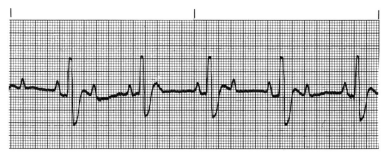

Mobitz II

Clinical Picture

- patient may notice slow rate
- slow rate may cause signs or symptoms of decreased cardiac output
- can only be diagnosed by EKG

Treatment

Field treatment of Mobitz II is aimed at improving conduction through the AV node. If the patient shows signs or symptoms of decreased cardiac output, atropine may improve AV conduction and increase the heart rate. If the use of atropine is unsuccessful, Isuprel may be necessary.

THIRD DEGREE AV BLOCK - COMPLETE HEART BLOCK

Etiology

In third degree AV block the SA node initiates impulses normally, but none of them is conducted through to the ventricles due to a complete block at the AV node. Therefore, the ventricles must be stimulated by either a junctional or ventricular escape mechanism or ventricular standstill will result. The upright P waves indicate normal atrial activity, but the QRS complexes have no relationship to the P waves as demonstrated by totally inconsistent PRI's and an occasional P wave occurring in the middle of a QRS. The inconsistent PRI and the presence of AV dissociation are keys in differentiating complete heart block from other heart blocks.

The QRS complexes may be normal or widened depending upon where the escape pacemaker originates. If the pacemaker is close to the junction, the rate will be 40–60 beats per minute and the QRS complex will be normal. If, however, the pacemaker arises lower in the bundle branches or Purkinje fibers, the rate will be 20–40 beats per minute and the QRS complex will be .12 seconds or greater.

Third degree heart block is most commonly caused by damage to the AV node, but can also result from drug overdose. This arrhythmia is considered life-threatening because the rate frequently reduces cardiac output and may lead to asystole.

Identifying Features

Rhythm	P–P regular; R–R regular
Rate	atrial rate usually normal; ventricular rate usually less than 40 beats/min, but may vary
P wave	normal and upright in Lead II; no relationship to QRS
PR interval	characteristically inconsistent; no relationship between P wave and QRS complex
QRS	less than .12 seconds if impulse is from the junction; .12 seconds or greater if impulse is from the ventricle

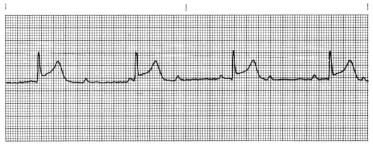

3rd-Degree Heart Block with a Junctional Escape Rhythm

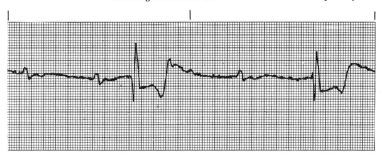

3rd-Degree Heart Block with a Ventricular Escape Rhythm

Clinical Picture

- patient may show signs or symptoms of decreased cardiac output and may lose consciousness
- very slow heart rate
- this arrhythmia can cause Stokes-Adams attacks (transient syncopal episodes associated with intermittent periods of first and third degree heart block)
- patient may be in congestive heart failure

Treatment

Field treatment is aimed at increasing the ventricular rate to improve cardiac output. If the escape rhythm originates in the junction it will usually respond to atropine. However, if the impulse originates in the ventricle, an Isuprel drip is indicated. Field treatment is merely supportive; treatment of choice for this arrhythmia is the in–hospital insertion of a pacemaker. Third degree heart block may be temporary or permanent, depending upon the extent of the damage to the AV node.

PREMATURE VENTRICULAR CONTRACTIONS

Etiology

In a premature ventricular contraction (PVC), an irritable focus within the ventricle initiates an impulse and overrides the normal pacemaker. The sinus node continues to fire but finds the ventricles refractory from the premature beat. Therefore, the P wave may be lost in the QRS or T wave. Due to the abnormal conduction through the ventricles, the QRS will be wide and bizarre (.12 seconds or greater). PVCs are usually followed by a fully compensatory pause unless retrograde conduction occurs, in which case the SA node can reset itself. Since PVCs are individual beats, the underlying arrhythmia must also be identified. The irritable focus within the ventricles may be caused by damage to the His-Purkinje system, hypoxia, acidosis, low potassium, congestive heart failure or digitalis toxicity.

Identifying Features

Rhythm	regular except for early beat
Rate	depends on the underlying rhythm
P wave	usually lost in QRS; occasionally may be seen in the T wave
PR interval	none
QRS	.12 seconds or greater; wide and bizarre. T wave is usually in opposite direction from QRS

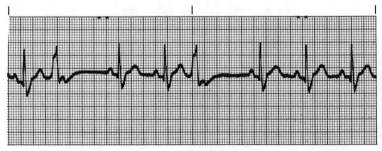

SR with Premature Ventricular Contractions

262

Clinical Picture

- most patients are aware of irregular pulse
- an apical or radial pulse will reveal a long pause following the premature beat

Treatment

PVCs are not always considered dangerous. The following list identifies circumstances in which PVCs should be considered dangerous and require treatment:

- greater than 6/min
- bigeminy and trigeminy
- coupling
- multifocal
- rapid succession of PVCs in a row
- "R on T" phenomenon
- any PVC in the presence of a myocardial infarction

The aim of treatment is to suppress the irritable focus within the ventricle. Lidocaine works quickly to decrease ventricular ectopics.

VENTRICULAR TACHYCARDIA

Etiology

Ventricular tachycardia (VT) is usually defined as three or more PVCs in a row. It may develop spontaneously, but is usually preceded by other signs of irritability such as PVCs. If P waves are present they will have no relationship to the QRS complexes; more commonly, P waves are not visible because they are hidden in the QRS complexes. Ventricular tachycardia is a form of AV dissociation, as the atria and ventricles beat independently of each other. Since the impulse arises outside of the normal conduction system, the QRS complex appears wide and bizarre and is .12 seconds or greater in duration. This rhythm is indicative of severe myocardial hypoxia or irritability and can advance very quickly to ventricular fibrillation. Because ventricular tachycardia causes a dramatic drop in cardiac output and progresses quickly to ventricular fibrillation, treatment must be initiated immediately.

Identifying Features

Rhythm	usually regular; may be *slightly* irregular
Rate	150–250 beats/min, may be slower
P wave	may be present or absent. If present, it has no relationship to QRS or is buried in QRS.
PR interval	none
QRS	wide and bizarre: .12 seconds or greater

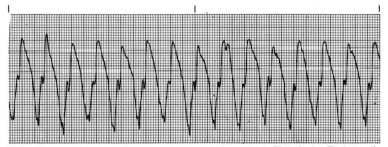

Ventricular Tachycardia

Clinical Picture

- if patient is conscious he is aware of rapid heart rate
- may develop signs or symptoms of decreased cardiac output
- cerebral anoxia may induce seizure
- peripheral pulses may be absent

Treatment

Field treatment is aimed at suppressing ventricular irritability. In a conscious patient, lidocaine will usually convert this arrhythmia. In a patient who is unconscious, or not perfusing, VT is best treated by defibrillating or cardioverting. Following conversion, lidocaine should be given to prevent recurrence. Ventricular irritability in the presence of chest pain is very dangerous and should be treated immediately.

VENTRICULAR FIBRILLATION

Etiology

In ventricular fibrillation (VF), many irritable foci initiate impulses in the ventricles causing a rapid, repetitive series of chaotic fibrillatory waves. These waves have no uniformity and are bizarre in configuration. There are no visible P waves or QRS complexes and the ventricles are completely ineffective as pumps. Poor electrode contact can create an electrical pattern very similar to VF. Therefore, be sure to check the patient's pulse before instituting treatment. The exact mechanism that triggers ventricular fibrillation is unknown, but it is often preceded by a PVC falling on the T wave.

Identifying Features

Rhythm
Rate
P wave } grossly chaotic with
PRI no discernible waves or complexes
QRS

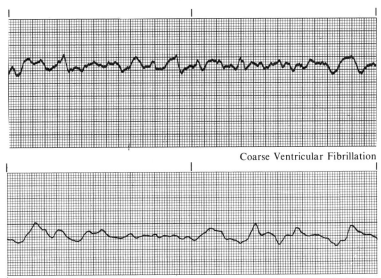

Coarse Ventricular Fibrillation

Fine Ventricular Fibrillation

Clinical Picture

- patient is unconscious and may convulse due to cerebral anoxia
- patient is clinically dead: there are no obtainable peripheral pulses, blood pressure, respirations, or heart sounds
- cyanosis and dilated pupils follow quickly

Treatment

Initiate CPR while preparing to defibrillate. In a witnessed arrest, defibrillation is the treatment of choice and should be done as quickly as possible to enhance the chances of conversion. In an unwitnessed arrest, sodium bicarbonate and Epinephrine should be given prior to defibrillation. Calcium chloride may be administered to help convert fine VF to coarse VF, thus making it more responsive to therapy. Once conversion has been accomplished, Lidocaine should be administered unless the resulting arrhythmia contraindicates its use.

IDIOVENTRICULAR (DYING HEART, AGONAL RHYTHM)

Etiology

In an idioventricular rhythm, the pacemaker function is taken over by the ventricles due to failure of the SA node and the AV junction to initiate impulses. This is the heart's final protective backup system. The impulses are initiated at a rate of less than 40 per minute, and conduction through the ventricles is abnormal causing a wider than normal QRS. Idioventricular rhythm can follow any severe medical condition such as MI, drowning, or trauma in which cardiac function is no longer effective. It is frequently the first rhythm found when assessing an arrested patient with a paddle check. Idioventricular or agonal rhythm commonly presents itself at some time during resuscitation when some definitive therapy has been administered. Very often the electrical activity is produced without any corresponding mechanical function or pulse.

Identifying Features

Rhythm   usually regular
Rate   less than 40 beats/min
P wave   if present, is not usually related to QRS
PR interval unable to measure
QRS   wide and bizarre; .12 seconds or greater

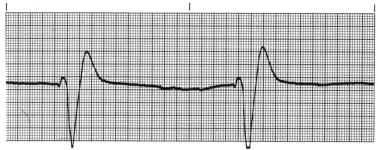

Idioventricular Rhythm

Clinical Picture

- if rate and perfusion are fairly good, patient may be awake, although sensorium will probably be altered
- if rate is low and perfusion is poor, the patient may have absent peripheral pulses, respirations, blood pressure, and heart sounds; patient is clinically dead

Treatment

This patient will probably require full resuscitation, and the arrhythmia should be treated immediately. Therapy is aimed at enhancing higher pacemaker sites and increasing heart rate. Once sodium bicarbonate is on board, Epinephrine, Isuprel, and calcium chloride should be given. Lidocaine is contraindicated in this ventricular arrhythmia since it may wipe out the protective mechanism and cause asystole.

ASYSTOLE AND VENTRICULAR STANDSTILL

Etiology

Asystole is a form of ventricular standstill wherein both the atria and the ventricles cease to contract because of absent or inadequate electrical stimulation. There are no P waves or QRS complexes on the EKG, thus creating a straight line. Ventricular standstill differs from asystole in that atrial conduction may continue, but ventricular conduction is absent. This produces an EKG with P waves but no QRS complexes. Both arrhythmias are considered nonviable, and will result in imminent death if not corrected immediately.

Identifying Features

Rhythm	no ventricular activity
Rate	no ventricular activity
P wave	absent in asystole, normal in ventricular standstill
PR interval	none
QRS	none

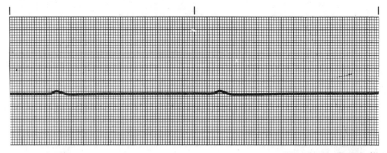

Ventricular Standstill

Clinical Picture

- patient is unconscious and may convulse due to cerebral anoxia
- no obtainable peripheral pulses, blood pressure, respirations, or heart sounds; patient is clinically dead
- can only be distinguished from VF by EKG
- cyanosis and dilated pupils follow quickly

Treatment

Begin CPR immediately and initiate drug therapy. Give sodium bicarbonate initially to correct acidosis. Follow this with Epinephrine and/or Isuprel and calcium chloride.

PACEMAKERS

Etiology

If the electrical system of the heart fails, it is possible to stimulate the myocardium by an external source. An electrode pacing wire is placed in either the atrium or ventricle and connected to a pulse generator which discharges electrical impulses at a given rate. Because the electrode is in direct contact with the heart muscle, this impulse stimulates myocardial contraction. The electrical stimulus is represented on the EKG by a spike or blip. Atrial pacemakers produce a pacemaker spike preceding the P wave which stimulates a QRS with normal conduction through the ventricles. Ventricular pacemakers produce a wide, or bizarre, QRS due to the initiation of the impulse below the bundle of His. At first glance a ventricular pacemaker rhythm looks just like VT, but the spikes preceding the QRS readily identify it. Ventricular pacemakers are used more commonly than atrial pacemakers because they bypass the AV junction which is frequently damaged by an MI. If the patient has a permanent pacemaker – as evidenced by a subcutaneous implant – but no pacemaker blips are visible, try another lead to see if they show any better. Two types of pacemakers are commonly seen:

Transthoracic pacemakers. During emergency situations, a thin-wire electrode can be passed through the chest wall to provide direct electrical stimulus to the myocardium. Once in place, a battery-powered pulse generator is attached and set at a sufficient rate to produce a viable rhythm.

Permanent pacemakers. Patients can be sent home with a pulse generator implanted in the subcutaneous tissue just below the skin. The electrode wires are attached to the endocardial or epicardial surface to provide the pacing stimulus.

Most pacemakers have a "demand" function. This means that the pulse generator is designed to sense the heart's contractions and discharges only if the heart actually needs it.

The EKG strip of a patient with a pacemaker should show either a sinus beat, or in its absence, a complex preceded by a pacemaker blip. Malfunctioning pacemakers can be identified by the absence of blips in a patient with a pacemaker, or by blips without a resultant QRS complex. A malfunctioning pacemaker is a serious condition because it leaves the patient to rely on his underlying cardiac function, which is usually a severe bradycardia or heart block.

Malfunctioning pacemakers can be caused by displacement of the catheter tip, a low or dead battery, perforation of the ventricular wall by the pacing electrode, or exposure to an unshielded microwave oven.

Identifying Features

Rhythm	regular when paced
Rate	depends on setting of pacemaker, usually normal
P wave	may be absent or present, no relationship to QRS
PR interval	unable to measure
QRS	wide and bizarre, impulse initiated in ventricle; characteristically preceded by a pacemaker spike

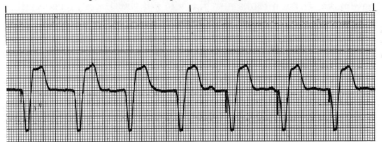

Functioning Pacemaker

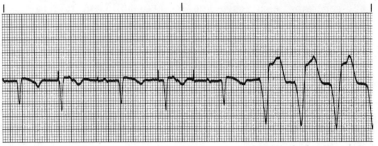

Malfunctioning Pacemaker

Clinical Features

- if the patient has a permanent pacemaker the battery will be seen as a protrusion under the skin
- will see pacemaker blip or spike on EKG monitor
- signs or symptoms of drop in cardiac output may occur depending upon the patient's underlying problem

Treatment

Pacemaker rhythms are only treated if they are malfunctioning. Very often severe bradycardias may result with a subsequent drop in cardiac output. If this occurs, treat the underlying arrhythmia by stimulating the heart with atropine, Isuprel, and/or Epinephrine and transport quickly for a medical evaluation.

FEATURES THAT COMPLICATE
INTERPRETATION

ABERRANCY

Aberrancy refers to abnormal conduction through the ventricles. This occurs because one bundle branch is still refractory while the other branch is ready to receive a stimulus. This prolongs conduction through the ventricles and thereby causes a wide, bizarre QRS very similar in appearance to a ventricular complex. Aberrancy has no clinical significance and cannot be conclusively diagnosed in the field. To spend time trying to differentiate between a supraventricular arrhythmia with aberrancy and a ventricular arrhythmia can delay treatment and cause patient death. Therefore, whenever you see a wide QRS, treat the patient as if the rhythm is ventricular until you have legitimate reason to think otherwise.

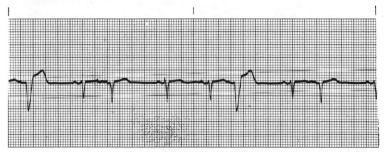

2 Aberrantly Conducted Beats

AV DISSOCIATION

AV dissociation is a term which is used to describe an arrhythmia, but is not a rhythm or diagnosis in itself. This term implies only that the atria and ventricles are functioning independently of each other. AV dissociation commonly occurs in third degree heart block, ventricular tachycardia, PVC, and junctional tachycardia.

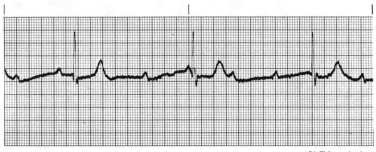

AV Dissociation

BUNDLE BRANCH BLOCK

This is not an arrhythmia but a ventricular conduction defect that may be present in any arrhythmia. The SA node is usually the pacemaker and conduction proceeds normally through the AV node to the Bundle of His. Since one bundle branch is blocked, the undamaged bundle conducts the impulse from the AV node to the Purkinje fibers of the ventricle it supplies. The impulse is finally conducted to the blocked ventricle by passing through the interventricular septum. This round-about path through the ventricles causes a wide or notched QRS complex, usually .12 seconds or greater in duration. This phenomenon may be caused by tissue damage resulting from an infarction or fibrotic scarring of the bundle itself. If both bundle branches become blocked, serious arrhythmias may result.

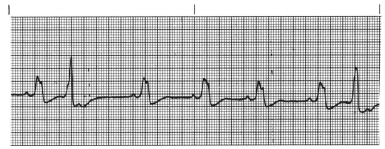

Bundle Branch Block

ELECTROMECHANICAL DISSOCIATION

Electromechanical dissociation is a condition wherein electrical activity is present in the heart but mechanical function is inadequate to sustain life. That is, the rhythm on the scope would be expected to produce a pulse, but no pulse is palpable in the patient. This condition can only be diagnosed by assessing the pulse while simultaneously looking at the EKG monitor. Electromechanical dissociation most commonly follows injury to the myocardium, as in cardiogenic shock or ventricular trauma. The patient is usually unconscious with no obtainable pulses or blood pressure. This patient will require full resuscitative measures as well as treatment specific for this condition. Treatment is aimed at improving the contractility of the heart muscle with calcium chloride. Epinephrine can be given concurrently to improve conduction and contractility.

ESCAPE MECHANISM

The heart has a built-in lifesaving mechanism that allows an impulse from the junction or the ventricle to escape and take over when higher pacing centers fail. This escape mechanism can take over for a single beat or for an entire rhythm. Escape beats can be differentiated from irritable premature contractions in that they come late in the cardiac cycle rather than early. Escape rhythms usually have a rate below 60 beats/min.

Escape beats and escape rhythms should not be suppressed; they should be stimulated. For this reason, lidocaine is contraindicated, and Atropine or Isuprel are more appropriate.

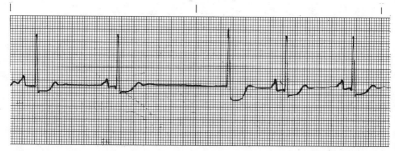

Junctional Escape Beat

ST ELEVATION AND ST DEPRESSION

ST elevation or ST depression may be an indication that the heart muscle has suffered insult as a result of coronary artery disease. Elevation of the ST segment is consistent with injury, while depression of the ST suggests ischemia.

Other possible causes of ST elevation include pericarditis or a ventricular aneurysm. A depressed ST segment may be a normal effect of digitalis.

ST changes are unreliable when seen on the field monitor but should not be ignored in a patient with chest pain.

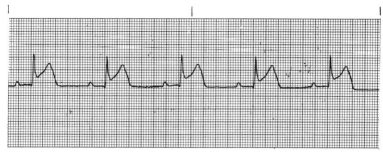

ST Elevation

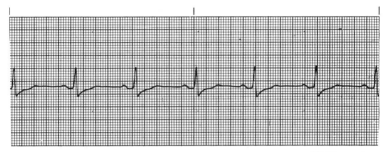

ST Depression

SELF-ASSESSMENT QUESTIONS

ARRHYTHMIAS

1. What is depolarization?
2. What is repolarization?
3. Define the properties of cardiac cells:

   a. contractility
   b. conductivity
   c. excitability
   d. automaticity
   e. rhythmicity
   f. refractoriness

4. Draw the normal conduction system.
5. Differentiate between the electrical and mechanical activities of the heart.
6. Identify the intrinsic rate for the SA node, AV junction and the ventricle.
7. Differentiate between escape and irritability.
8. Explain the relative refractory period. When does it occur on the EKG? Why is it called vulnerable?
9. Discuss retrograde conduction.
10. How many seconds are represented by one small box on EKG paper? One large box?
11. List three ways to calculate heart rate.
12. What is the normal PR interval?
13. What is the normal QRS interval?
14. What does the P wave represent?
15. What does the QRS complex represent?
16. What does the T wave represent?
17. What does the PR interval represent?
18. List the five steps in analyzing an arrhythmia.
19. Draw and label a normal EKG complex (include P, Q, R, S, T, PR interval, QRS, ST).
20. Define tachycardia.
21. Define bradycardia.
22. List two or three distinguishing characteristics of each of the following

arrhythmias and relate this to the conduction system:

a. Sinus arrhythmia
b. PAC
c. WAP
d. SA block/SA arrest
e. Atrial tachycardia
f. Atrial tachycardia with block
g. Atrial flutter
h. Atrial fibrillation
i. Junctional rhythm
j. Accelerated junctional rhythm
k. Junctional tachycardia
l. PJC
m. First degree AV block
n. Mobitz I
o. Mobitz II
p. Third degree AV block
q. PVC
r. Escape ventricular beat
s. Ventricular tachycardia
t. Ventricular fibrillation
u. Idioventricular
v. Asystole
w. Pacemaker rhythm
x. Normal sinus rhythm
y. Sinus tachycardia
z. Sinus bradycardia
aa. Supraventricular tachycardia
bb. Ventricular standstill

23. Explain electromechanical dissociation.
24. Explain AV dissociation.
25. List two arrhythmias in which AV dissociation is present.
26. When are arrhythmias treated in the field?
27. List three methods of field treatment for supraventricular tachycardias.
28. What are the two drugs used for the treatment of bradycardias?
29. In the presence of bradycardia, which drug is used in the treatment of PVCs?

30. Under what circumstances should PVCs be considered dangerous and in need of treatment?
31. What is the drug of choice for PVCs?
32. What is the drug of choice for treatment of complete heart block?
33. What is the treatment for ventricular tachycardia:
    a. in a conscious patient?
    b. in a pulseless patient?
34. What is the treatment for ventricular fibrillation?
35. What is the treatment for asystole?
36. Why is a supraventricular tachycardia dangerous in the presence of a myocardial infarction?
37. What is the treatment of electromechanical dissociation?
38. What is the treatment of idioventricular rhythm?
39. How do you treat ventricular escape beats?
40. Why must CPR be maintained during treatment of life-threatening arrhythmias?
41. How is a malfunctioning pacemaker treated in the field?

SELF-ASSESSMENT SITUATIONS

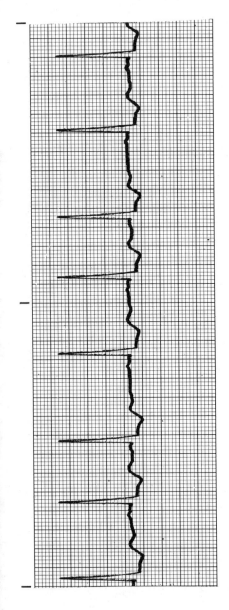

1.

SITUATION: EKG of a 53 year old male who states he has had the flu for several days and wants to go to the hospital. Vital signs are stable.

INTERPRETATION:

TREATMENT:

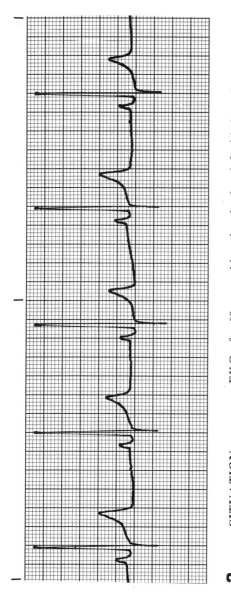

2.

SITUATION: EKG of a 60 year old male who has left sided weakness and difficulty speaking. Blood pressure is 160/110; respirations are 24 and regular.

INTERPRETATION:

TREATMENT:

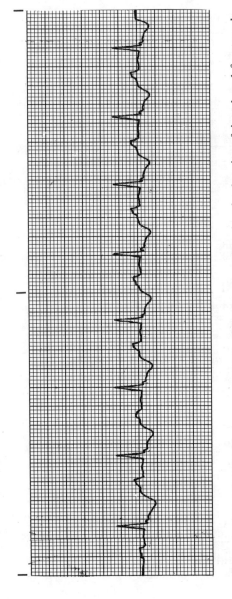

3.

SITUATION: EKG of a 62 year old male who has just fainted and fractured his hip. Blood pressure is 110/70.

INTERPRETATION:

TREATMENT:

Self-Assessment

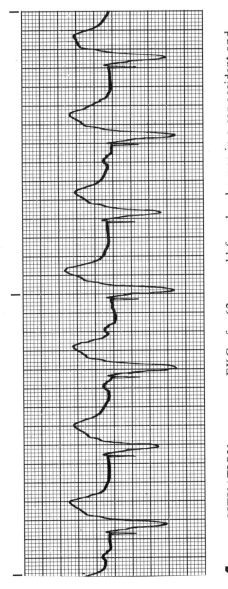

4.

SITUATION: EKG of a 62 year old female who was in a car accident and has a broken wrist. Vital signs are stable.

INTERPRETATION:

TREATMENT:

287

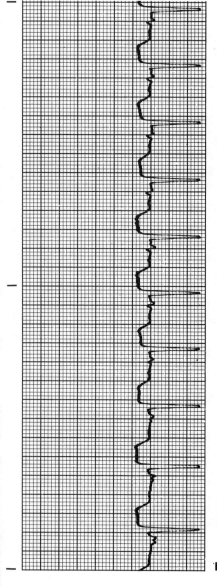

5.

SITUATION: EKG of a 46 year old woman complaining of nausea, diaphoresis, indigestion and shortness of breath. Her blood pressure is 126/92; respirations 22.

INTERPRETATION:

TREATMENT:

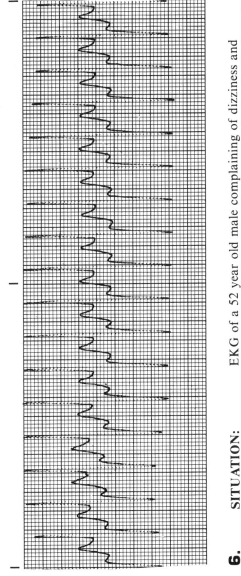

6.

SITUATION: EKG of a 52 year old male complaining of dizziness and palpitations. Blood pressure is 90/60. He is slightly diaphoretic and somewhat dyspneic.

INTERPRETATION:

TREATMENT:

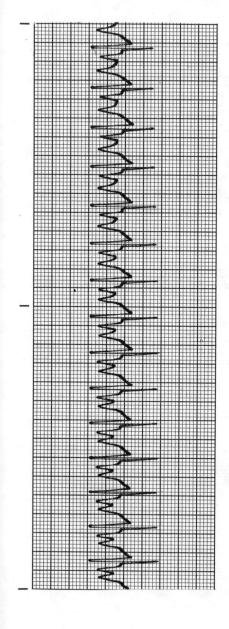

7. **SITUATION:** EKG of a 45 year old male who experienced an MI one month ago. He is now complaining of pain upon inspiration, hemeoptysis and severe dyspnea. Blood pressure is 120/90; respirations 32.

INTERPRETATION:
TREATMENT:

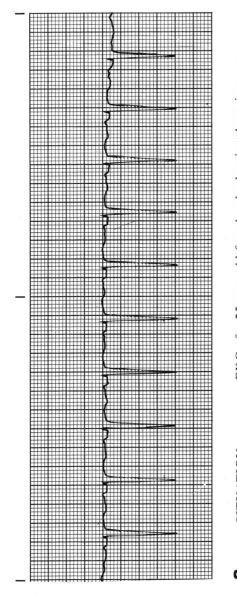

8.

SITUATION: EKG of a 25 year old female who has just been in a car accident. She has no apparent injuries and her vital signs are stable.

INTERPRETATION:

TREATMENT:

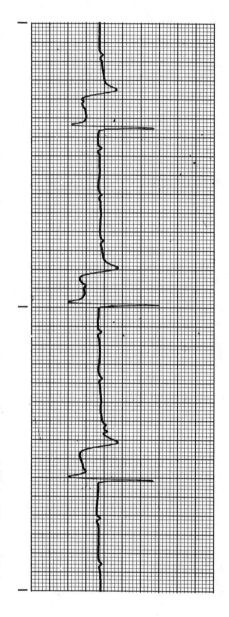

9.

SITUATION: EKG of an 89 year old female who was found unconscious by her housekeeper. She is now awake but disoriented. Her blood pressure is 90/60.

INTERPRETATION:

TREATMENT:

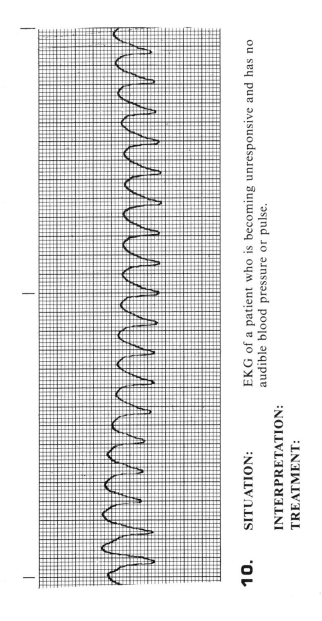

10. **SITUATION:** EKG of a patient who is becoming unresponsive and has no audible blood pressure or pulse.

INTERPRETATION:

TREATMENT:

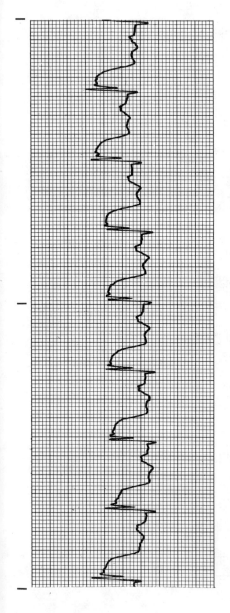

11. SITUATION: EKG of a 45 year old male complaining of severe, crushing, substernal chest pain of two hours duration. He is short of breath and nauseated. Blood pressure is 140/90.

INTERPRETATION:

TREATMENT:

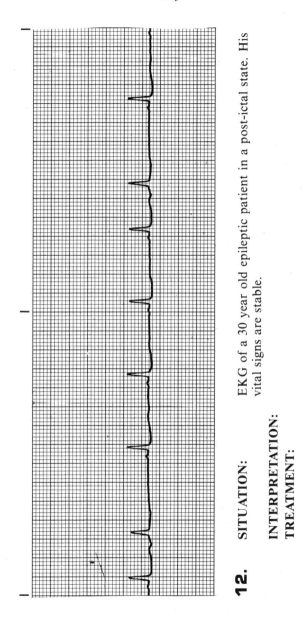

12. **SITUATION:** EKG of a 30 year old epileptic patient in a post-ictal state. His vital signs are stable.

INTERPRETATION:

TREATMENT:

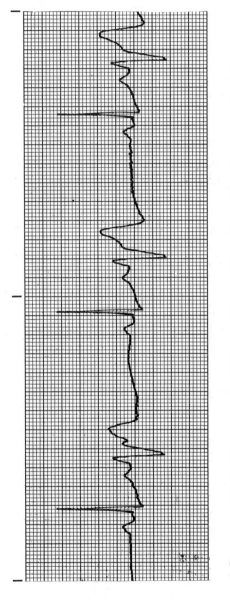

13.

SITUATION: EKG of a 72 year old patient with a history of heart disease who is on Digoxin orally. He is complaining of dizziness and has a palpable radial pulse of 30. His blood pressure is 100/70.

INTERPRETATION:

TREATMENT:

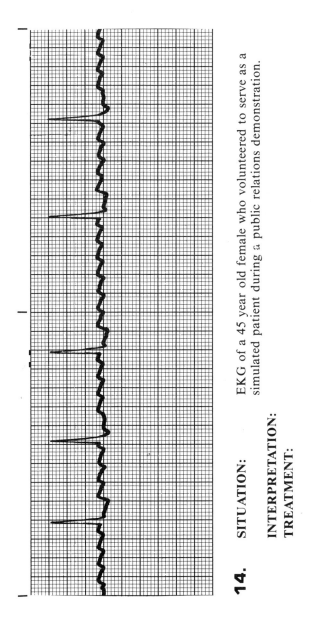

14.

SITUATION: EKG of a 45 year old female who volunteered to serve as a simulated patient during a public relations demonstration.

INTERPRETATION:

TREATMENT:

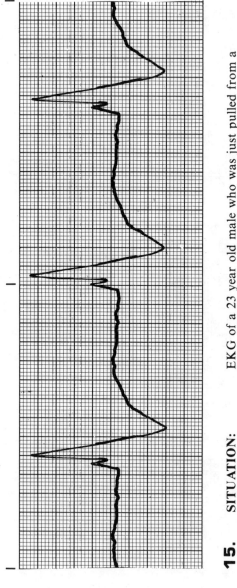

15. SITUATION: EKG of a 23 year old male who was just pulled from a swimming pool. He is unconscious, pulseless, and apneic.

INTERPRETATION:

TREATMENT:

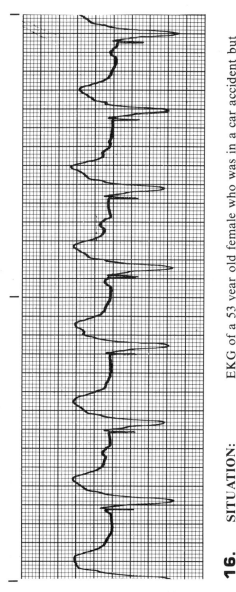

16.

SITUATION: EKG of a 53 year old female who was in a car accident but complains of gastric distress and says she has been vomiting dark coffee-ground material. Her vital signs are stable, although she appeared in moderate distress.

INTERPRETATION:
TREATMENT:

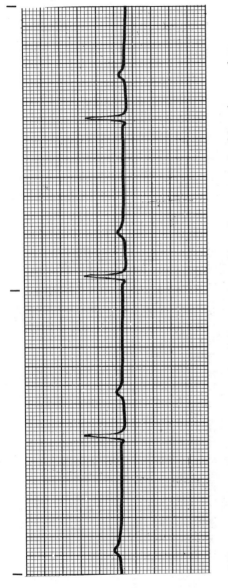

17.

SITUATION: EKG of a 27 year old male, suspected of heroin overdose. Blood pressure is 90/60; respirations are 8 and shallow.

INTERPRETATION:

TREATMENT:

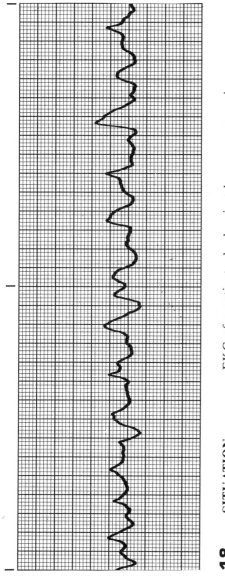

18. **SITUATION:** EKG of a patient who has just become unconscious, pulseless, and apneic.

INTERPRETATION:
TREATMENT:

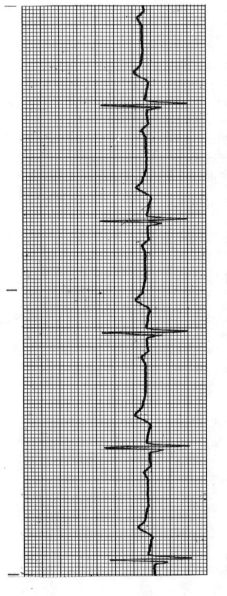

19. **SITUATION:** EKG of a 65 year old male who has had a pacemaker for two years. He is complaining of feeling dizzy. Blood pressure is 80/60.

INTERPRETATION:

TREATMENT:

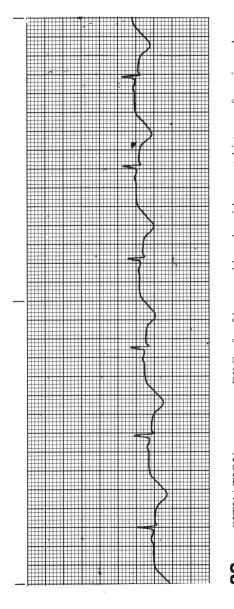

20.

SITUATION: EKG of a 51 year old male with a past history of angina who is now complaining of mild chest pain after jogging. His pain has lasted 10–15 minutes. His blood pressure is 150/94.

INTERPRETATION:

TREATMENT:

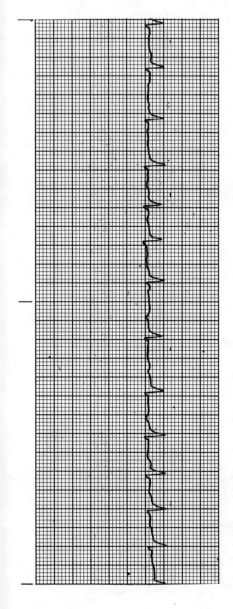

21. SITUATION: EKG of 45 year old female who had valve surgery three years ago and is now complaining of palpitations and mild shortness of breath. Lungs have rales in the bases. Blood pressure is 140/90 and respirations are 24.

INTERPRETATION:

TREATMENT:

304

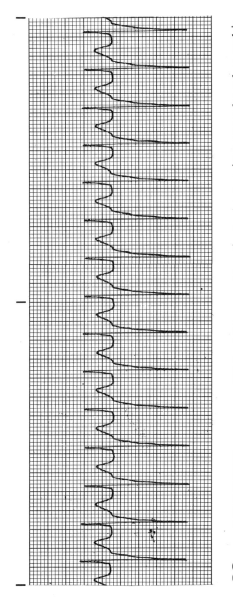

22.

SITUATION: EKG of 29 year old patient who was just stung by a bee and is complaining of severe respiratory difficulty. His vital signs are blood pressure 90/60, respirations 36.

INTERPRETATION:

TREATMENT:

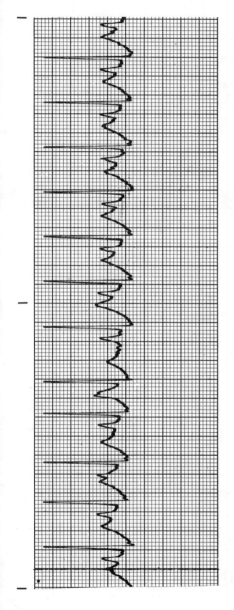

23. **SITUATION:** EKG of a 19 year old victim of a motorcycle accident suffering a fractured femur with arterial bleeding. Blood pressure is 100/70.

INTERPRETATION:
TREATMENT:

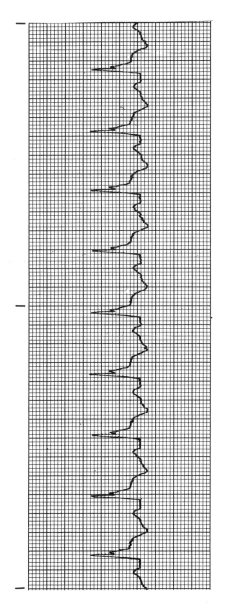

24. **SITUATION:** EKG of a 62 year old male who is experiencing a slight heaviness in the chest. He has a history of atherosclerosis. Vital signs are stable and the lungs are clear.

INTERPRETATION:

TREATMENT:

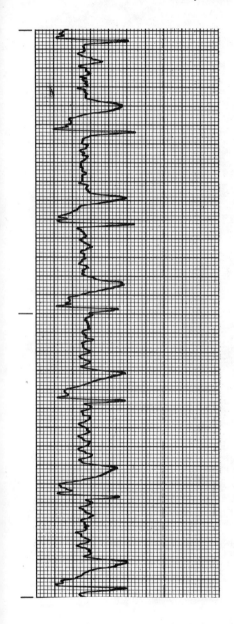

25.   **SITUATION:**   EKG of a 55 year old female who was in a car accident. Her only complaint is soreness across the precordium from where her chest hit the steering wheel. Her vital signs are stable and breath sounds are clear bilaterally.

INTERPRETATION:

TREATMENT:

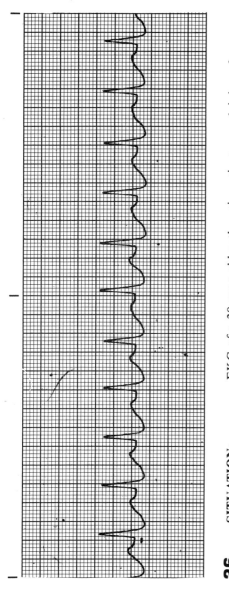

26. **SITUATION:** EKG of a 38 year old asthmatic patient complaining of severe dyspnea and has wheezes bilaterally. Vital signs are blood pressure 110/70, respirations 32 and shallow.

INTERPRETATION:

TREATMENT:

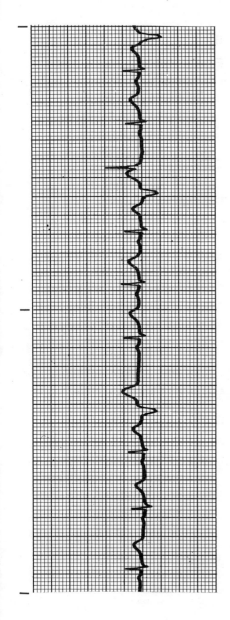

27.

SITUATION: EKG of a 46 year old male who quit taking his Pronestyl at home and is now complaining of palpitations. Vital signs are stable.

INTERPRETATION:

TREATMENT:

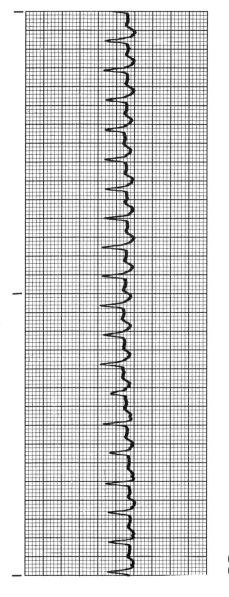

28. **SITUATION:** EKG of a 54 year old female who presents with cool, clammy skin, is diaphoretic, and has a decreased level of consciousness. Her blood pressure is 80/50.

INTERPRETATION:

TREATMENT:

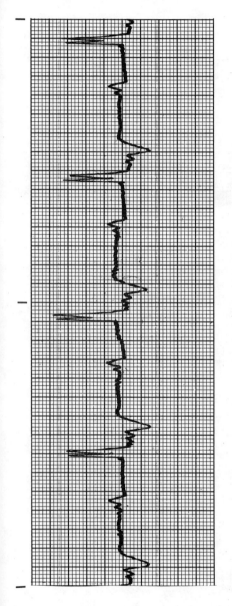

29. **SITUATION:** EKG of an 85 year old male complaining of dizziness. His blood pressure is 90/60.

INTERPRETATION:

TREATMENT:

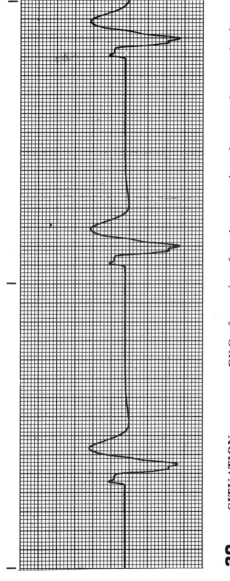

30. SITUATION: EKG of a patient found unconscious in a rest home, who is now pulseless, and apneic.

INTERPRETATION:
TREATMENT:

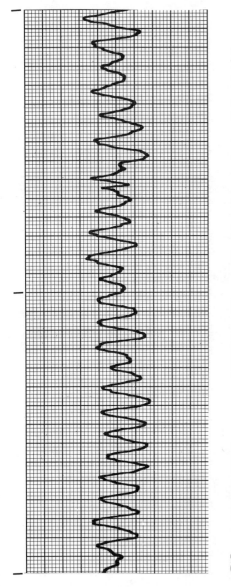

31. SITUATION: EKG of a 25 year old male who was just pulled out of the ocean by a lifeguard. He is pulseless and apneic.

INTERPRETATION:

TREATMENT:

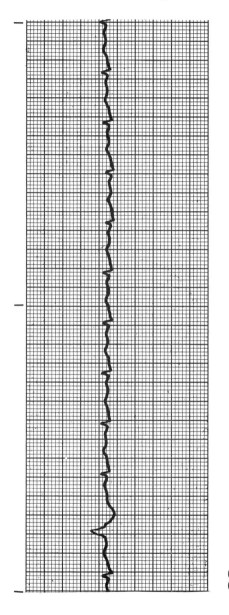

32.

SITUATION: EKG of a patient who was bitten less than 10 minutes ago by a rattlesnake. He is complaining of pain at the site on his leg. His blood pressure is 130/80, respirations 28 and shallow.

INTERPRETATION:

TREATMENT:

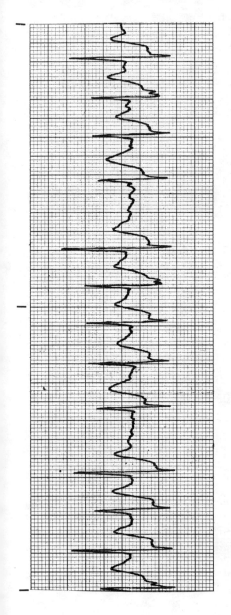

33.

SITUATION: EKG of a 64 year old male who has a history of heart disease. He is complaining of burning upon urination and colicky flank pain. Blood pressure 120/80.

INTERPRETATION:

TREATMENT:

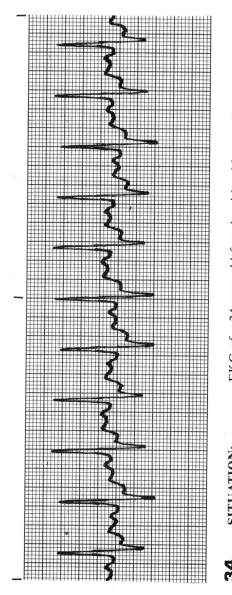

34.

SITUATION: EKG of a 34 year old female with a history of psychiatric problems who is hysterical and complaining that she can't breathe. She has tingling in her fingertips and a blood pressure of 130/70. Respirations are 32 and shallow. She has no history of heart or lung disease.

INTERPRETATION:

TREATMENT:

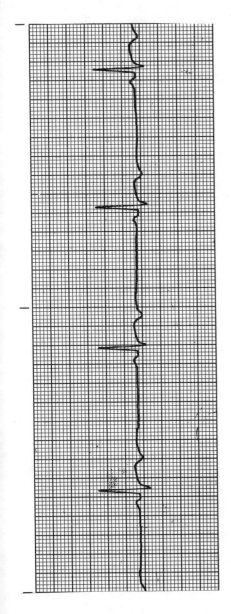

35.   SITUATION: EKG of a 28 year old male working at an excavation site when a sand hill caved in on him and covered him completely. When he was pulled out, he was cyanotic. His blood pressure is now 90/60.

INTERPRETATION:

TREATMENT:

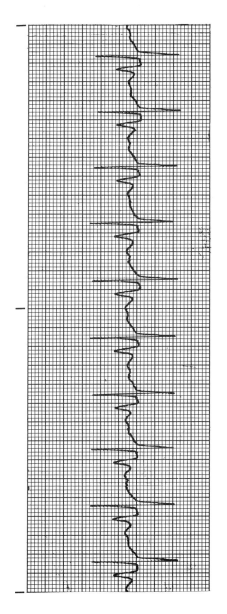

36.

SITUATION: EKG of a patient with chronic lung disease who is complaining of dyspnea and has wheezes on expiration. He is diaphoretic and pale. His blood pressure is 100/70, respirations are 32 and shallow.

INTERPRETATION:

TREATMENT:

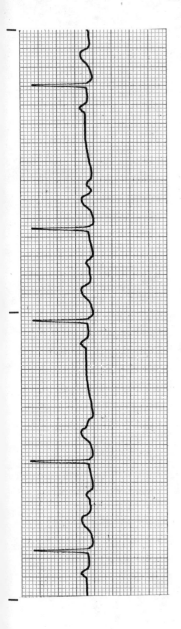

37. **SITUATION:** EKG of a 36 year old female who is complaining of severe substernal pressure radiating down both arms. She is cool and diaphoretic. Her blood pressure is 100/60.

INTERPRETATION:

TREATMENT:

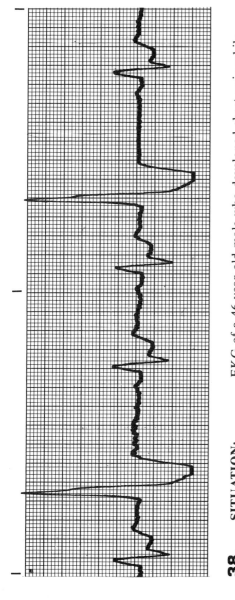

38. SITUATION: EKG of a 46 year old male who developed chest pain while mowing his lawn. It has lasted for 30 minutes and has continued despite resting. Blood pressure is 140/90. He has no history of prior heart disease.

INTERPRETATION:

TREATMENT:

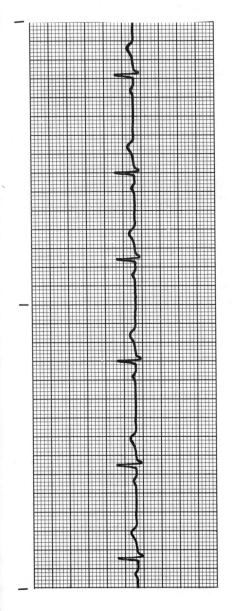

39. SITUATION: EKG of a 3 year old child who was trapped in an old refrigerator for two hours and has been resuscitated by his father. Vital signs are now stable.

INTERPRETATION:
TREATMENT:

322

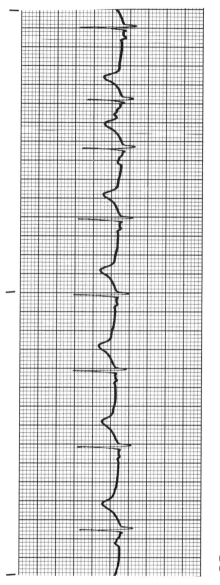

40.

SITUATION: EKG of a 42 year old male who has just attempted suicide by taking 50 Valium tablets. He is lethargic but his vital signs are stable. Estimated time of arrival at the hospital is 45 minutes.

INTERPRETATION:

TREATMENT:

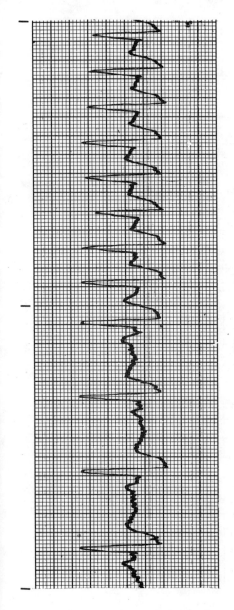

41.

SITUATION: EKG of a 65 year old female who is complaining of recurrent shortness of breath and palpitations. Vital signs are stable.

INTERPRETATION:

TREATMENT:

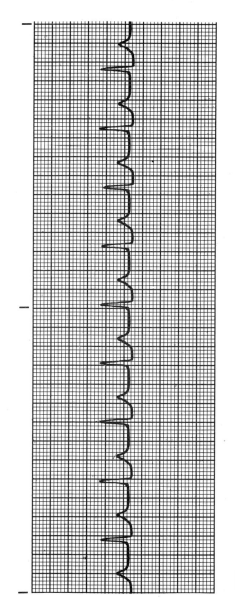

42.

SITUATION: EKG of a 19 year old male who has just been in a motorcycle accident and has sustained a head injury. His blood pressure is 140/84 and respirations are 14 and shallow. There are no other apparent injuries.

INTERPRETATION:

TREATMENT:

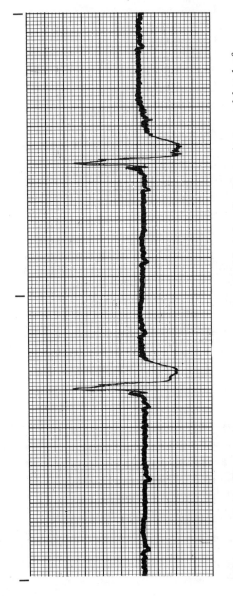

43. SITUATION: EKG of a 75 year old male who has a decreased level of consciousness. His blood pressure and respirations are unobtainable.

INTERPRETATION:
TREATMENT:

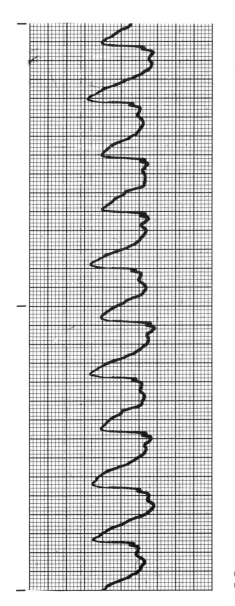

44. **SITUATION:** EKG of a 52 year old male complaining of severe crushing substernal chest pain with radiation down both arms that has lasted for 30 minutes. He is diaphoretic, cool and clammy. His blood pressure is 90/60 and respirations are 24.

INTERPRETATION:

TREATMENT:

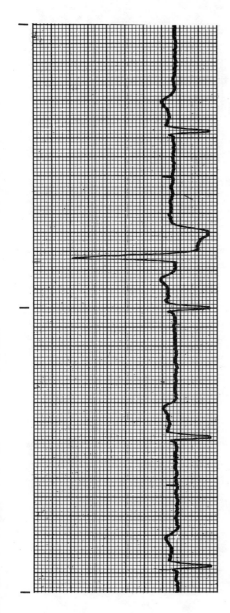

45.

SITUATION: EKG of a 65 year old female who collapsed in a restaurant. Her blood pressure is 100/72.

INTERPRETATION:

TREATMENT:

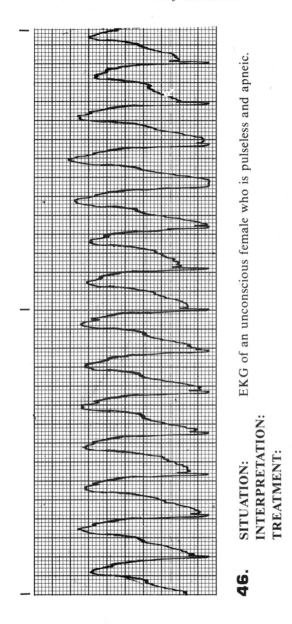

46.

SITUATION: EKG of an unconscious female who is pulseless and apneic.

INTERPRETATION:

TREATMENT:

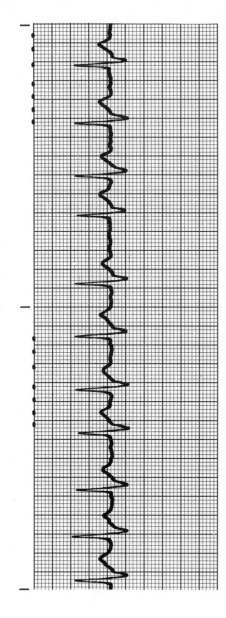

47. **SITUATION:** EKG of a 53 year old female just pulled out of a structure fire. She has sustained second and third degree burns to 45 percent of her body. Blood pressure is 136/80 and respirations are 24 and easy. She is alert, complaining of severe pain and has no other injuries.

INTERPRETATION:

TREATMENT:

330

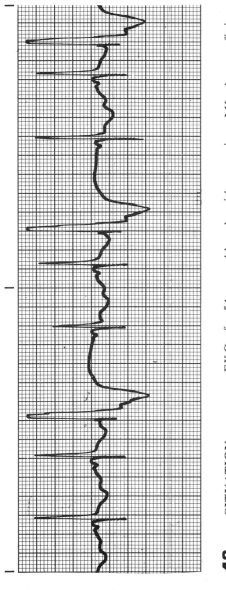

48.

SITUATION: EKG of a 54 year old male with a previous MI who was fixing an electrical outlet in his home. He was shocked and temporarily lost consciousness. He is now alert and his vital signs are stable.

INTERPRETATION:

TREATMENT:

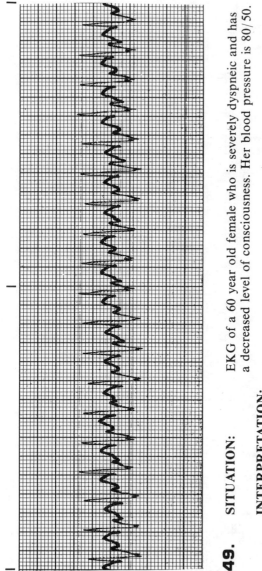

49.

SITUATION: EKG of a 60 year old female who is severely dyspneic and has a decreased level of consciousness. Her blood pressure is 80/50.

INTERPRETATION:

TREATMENT:

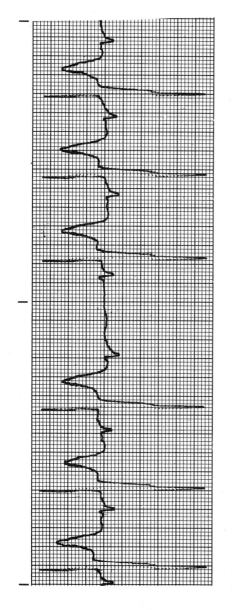

50. SITUATION: EKG of a 61 year old male complaining of heaviness in his chest which has persisted for one hour. He has a blood pressure of 130/70 and normal respirations.

INTERPRETATION:

TREATMENT:

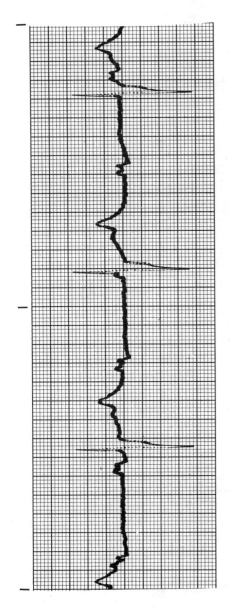

51. **SITUATION:** EKG of a 73 year old male who has been feeling light-headed, and has now fainted. Although unconscious, he responds to painful stimuli. His blood pressure is 90/60, and respirations are 10/min.

INTERPRETATION:

TREATMENT:

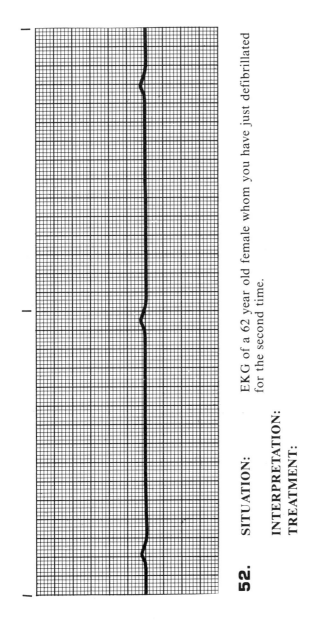

52.

SITUATION: EKG of a 62 year old female whom you have just defibrillated for the second time.

INTERPRETATION:

TREATMENT:

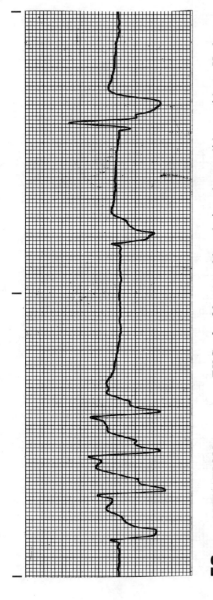

53.

SITUATION: EKG of a 20 year old male in a hang-glider accident. He has no palpable pulse, blood pressure, or spontaneous respirations.

INTERPRETATION:

TREATMENT:

336

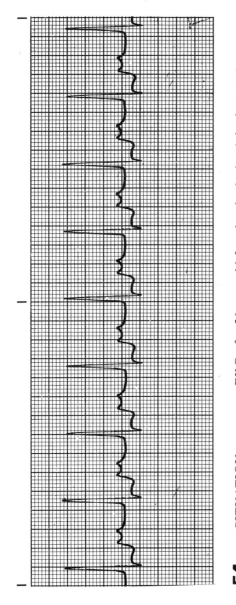

54. **SITUATION:** EKG of a 56 year old female who had palpitations and dizziness 15 minutes prior to your arrival. She is conscious, coherent and appears stable at this time. She had a mild heart attack one year ago and is taking Digoxin. Her blood pressure is 138/80, and respirations are 18/min.

INTERPRETATION:

TREATMENT:

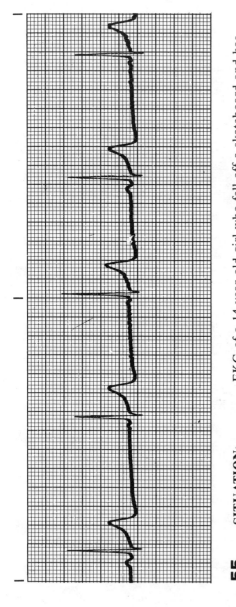

55. **SITUATION:** EKG of a 14 year old girl who fell off a skateboard and has a severe laceration of her left knee with no other apparent injuries. Her blood pressure is 120/80. Respirations are normal.

INTERPRETATION:

TREATMENT:

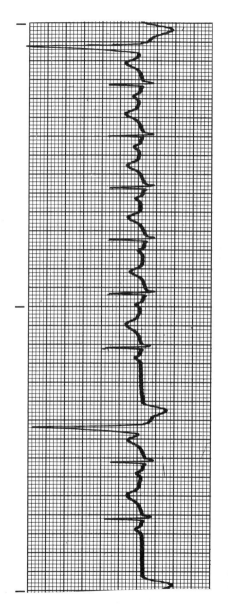

56. **SITUATION:** EKG of a 58 year old female suffering from chronic lung disease. She called you because she ran out of oxygen. Her vital signs are fairly stable although she appears in mild distress.

INTERPRETATION:
TREATMENT:

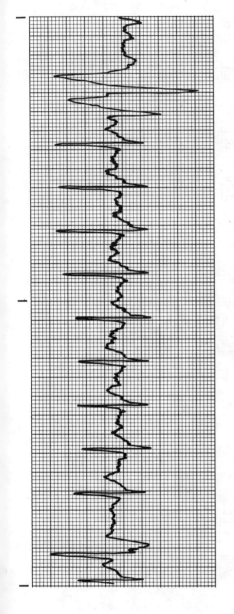

57. SITUATION: EKG of a 54 year old male who had an MI six months ago, and is now complaining of severe crushing chest pain. Just after you apply oxygen and start the IV he becomes less responsive and cyanotic. His blood pressure drops from 124/80 to 80/60.

INTERPRETATION:

TREATMENT:

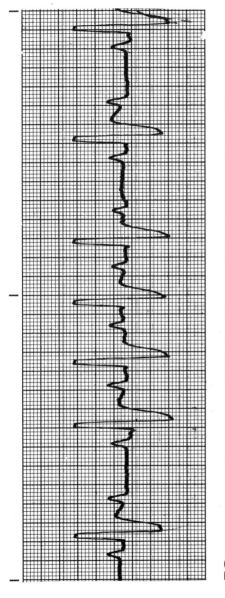

58.

SITUATION: EKG of a 72 year old female in a physician's office complaining of substernal chest pain. The pain has persisted for the past two hours and has increased in intensity. She is slightly diaphoretic and anxious. Her blood pressure is 138/76, and her respirations are 28 and full.

INTERPRETATION:

TREATMENT:

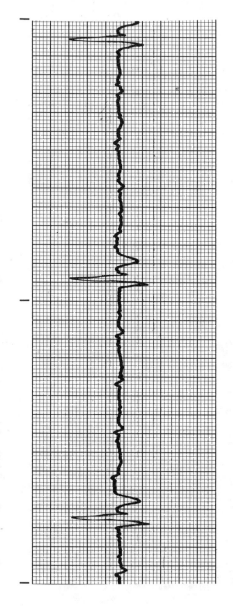

59.

SITUATION: EKG of an elderly man found unconscious, pulseless, and apneic on a golf course. No vital signs are obtainable.

INTERPRETATION:

TREATMENT:

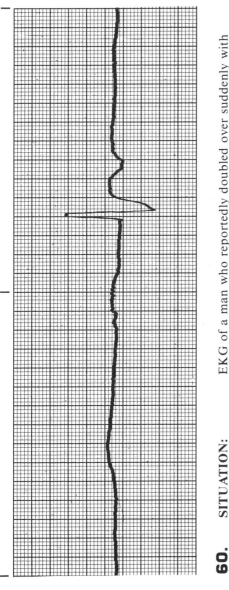

60. **SITUATION:** EKG of a man who reportedly doubled over suddenly with excruciating knife-like pain in his abdomen with radiation to his back. He then collapsed on the floor and is now pulseless and apneic.

INTERPRETATION:

TREATMENT:

343

ANSWERS TO SELF-ASSESSMENT SITUATIONS

1. Interpretation: Sinus rhythm with PACs.
   Treatment: Oxygen. Watch for increase in number of PACs.
2. Interpretation: Sinus bradycardia.
   Treatment: Oxygen and IV TKO.
3. Interpretation: Sinus rhythm with a first degree heart block, depressed ST segment and inverted T wave.
   Treatment: Oxygen, IV (RL or NS) TKO. Watch closely for progression into third degree heart block; stabilize the hip
4. Interpretation: Pacemaker rhythm with good capture.
   Treatment: Splint wrist. Rhythm does not require treatment.
5. Interpretation: Wandering atrial pacemaker with deep Q waves and elevated ST segment.
   Treatment: Oxygen, IV TKO, morphine. Consider prophylactic lidocaine.
6. Interpretation: Supraventricular tachycardia.
   Treatment: Oxygen, IV TKO, possibly Valsalva's maneuver and/or CSM. If no response, may try Inderal or digitalis. Consider cardioversion as a last resort.
7. Interpretation: Sinus tachycardia.
   Treatment: Oxygen; IV TKO, prompt transport.
8. Interpretation: Sinus tachycardia.
   Treatment: No treatment necessary.
9. Interpretation: Complete heart block with a junctional escape rhythm.
   Treatment: Oxygen; IV TKO; atropine; Isuprel.
10. Interpretation: Ventricular tachycardia.
    Treatment: Begin CPR; oxygen; IV TKO; cardiovert or defibrillate. Follow with lidocaine bolus and drip.
11. Interpretation: Sinus rhythm with borderline first degree heart block and elevated ST segment.
    Treatment: Oxygen; IV TKO; morphine sulfate for pain. Watch for further blocks, consider prophylactic lidocaine.
12. Interpretation: Sinus rhythm with PJCs.
    Treatment: High-flow oxygen; IV TKO; transport.

13. Interpretation: Sinus bradycardia with borderline first degree heart block and begeminy of PVCs.
    Treatment: Oxygen; IV TKO; atropine to increase heart rate. If PVCs persist after rate is increased, may need to treat with lidocaine bolus and drip. Watch closely and transport.
14. Interpretation: Atrial flutter with a variable response.
    Treatment: No treatment necessary.
15. Interpretation: Idioventricular rhythm.
    Treatment: Oxygen with positive pressure ventilation; CPR; sodium bicarbonate, Isuprel, Epinephrine, calcium chloride; nasogastric tube.
16. Interpretation: Paced rhythm.
    Treatment: Oxygen, IV (RL or NS), monitor vital signs closely.
17. Interpretation: Junctional rhythm.
    Treatment: Oxygen; assist ventilations; IV TKO; Narcan.
18. Interpretation: Coarse ventricular fibrillation.
    Treatment: CPR; ventilate; IV TKO; give sodium bicarbonate and Epinephrine and defibrillate. After conversion, follow with Lidocaine bolus and drip.
19. Interpretation: Mobitz II heart block with 2:1 conduction.
    Treatment: Oxygen; IV TKO; atropine, Isuprel; transport for insertion of a new pacemaker.
20. Interpretation: Sinus rhythm with depressed ST segment and inverted T wave.
    Treatment: Oxygen; IV TKO; nitroglycerin for chest pain.
21. Interpretation: Atrial fibrillation (rapid ventricular response).
    Treatment: Oxygen; IV TKO; morphine, Lasix. Consider rotating tourniquet and/or Aminophylline if condition warrants it.
22. Interpretation: Supraventricular tachycardia.
    Treatment: Oxygen; IV TKO. Treat the allergic reaction with Epinephrine SC and Benadryl. Rhythm should subside as patient's condition improves.
23. Interpretation: Sinus tachycardia with PAC's.
    Treatment: Oxygen; control the bleeding; IV RL, for

fluid replacement; splint the fracture.
Rhythm should subside as patient's
condition improves.

24. Interpretation: Sinus rhythm with borderline first degree
    heart block, bundle branch block, elevated
    ST segment and inverted T wave.
    Treatment: Oxygen; IV TKO; morphine, watch for
    further block. Consider prophylactic
    lidocaine.

25. Interpretation: Atrial flutter with elevated ST and inverted
    T wave.
    Treatment: Oxygen; IV TKO, monitor closely and
    transport.

26. Interpretation: Junctional tachycardia.
    Treatment: Oxygen; IV TKO; Isuprel Inhalant, Epine-
    phrine SC, or Aminophylline. The
    arrhythmia should subside as patient's
    condition improves.

27. Interpretation: Sinus tachycardia with frequent unifocal
    PVCs.
    Treatment: Oxygen; IV TKO; if PVCs persist,
    lidocaine, bolus and drip.

28. Interpretation: Supraventricular tachycardia.
    Treatment: Oxygen; IV TKO; Valsalva's maneuver;
    CSM; Inderal or Digoxin; cardioversion if
    necessary.

29. Interpretation: Mobitz II heart block, 2:1 conduction,
    bundle branch block.
    Treatment: Oxygen; IV TKO; atropine. Watch for
    further block.

30. Interpretation: Idioventricular rhythm.
    Treatment: CPR; ventilate; sodium bicarbonate,
    Isuprel, Epinephrine, calcium chloride.

31. Interpretation: Coarse ventricular fibrillation.
    Treatment: CPR, ventilate with positive pressure,
    IV TKO, sodium bicarbonate, Epinephrine,
    defibrillate, nasogastric tube.

32. Interpretation: Sinus tachycardia with one PVC.
    Treatment: Oxygen high flow, constricting band above
    the bite, cool packs around the site, lower
    the extremity and prevent movement, IV
    TKO, incise and suction the wound if
    ordered. Watch for increase in frequency of
    PVCs.

33. Interpretation: Atrial fibrillation.
    Treatment: IV TKO. No treatment of the atrial fibrillation is required at present as the patient is tolerating the arrhythmia.
34. Interpretation: Sinus tachycardia.
    Treatment: Calm patient down, have her breathe into a paper bag, possibly IV TKO as a precautionary measure.
35. Interpretation: Sinus bradycardia.
    Treatment: High flow oxygen, assist ventilations, IV TKO, sodium bicarbonate; atropine if heart rate does not increase from other treatment.
36. Interpretation: Borderline sinus tachycardia.
    Treatment: Low flow oxygen, IV TKO, Isuprel inhalant, Aminophylline, or Epinephrine SC.
37. Interpretation: Wenckebach (Mobitz I).
    Treatment: High flow oxygen, IV TKO, morphine for chest pain, watch for further heart block. May need atropine.
38. Interpretation: Borderline sinus bradycardia with first degree heart block, bundle branch block and PVCs.
    Treatment: High flow oxygen, IV TKO, nitroglycerine or morphine for chest pain. Consider atropine to increase the heart rate; if the PVCs still persist with an increased heart rate, may need to give lidocaine.
39. Interpretation: Sinus arrhythmia.
    Treatment: High flow oxygen and IV TKO.
40. Interpretation: Wandering atrial pacemaker with a PAC.
    Treatment: Oxygen, IV TKO. Narcan to determine if any narcotics have been taken. Due to the long transport time, may insert a nasogastric tube and begin saline irrigations. Position and watch closely for vomiting and aspiration. Have suction available.
41. Interpretation: Sinus rhythm going into PAT, bundle branch block.
    Treatment: Oxygen, IV TKO, check for signs or symptoms of CHF, watch closely for drop in cardiac output; if this occurs, may need Valsalva's maneuver, CSM, or drugs.
42. Interpretation: Accelerated junctional rhythm.

	Treatment:	High flow oxygen, may need to assist respirations, IV TKO, prompt transport.
43.	Interpretation:	Complete heart block with an escape ventricular rhythm.
	Treatment:	Assist ventilations with high flow oxygen, CPR, IV TKO, sodium bicarbonate, Isuprel, Epinephrine, and calcium chloride.
44.	Interpretation:	Borderline sinus tachycardia with pronounced ST elevation.
	Treatment:	High flow oxygen, IV TKO, morphine for pain, watch for ectopics. Consider prophylactic lidocaine.
45.	Interpretation:	Malfunctioning pacemaker with underlying junctional rhythm with a PVC.
	Treatment:	Oxygen, IV TKO, atropine, transport for insertion of a new pacemaker.
46.	Interpretation:	Ventricular tachycardia.
	Treatment:	CPR, cardiovert or defibrillate, IVC TKO, may need sodium bicarbonate. If the rhythm converts with countershock, treat the underlying arrhythmia and administer lidocaine.
47.	Interpretation:	Atrial fibrillation (rapid ventricular response).
	Treatment:	High flow oxygen, IV RL for fluid replacement. Keep warm and cover burn, administer morphine in small increments IV push for pain if necessary.
48.	Interpretation:	Accelerated junctional rhythm with trigeminy of PVCs.
	Treatment:	Oxygen, IV TKO, lidocaine bolus and drip, check for associated injuries.
49.	Interpretation:	Atrial tachycardia with bundle branch block.
	Treatment:	Oxygen, IV TKO, Valsalva's maneuver, CSM, digitalis or Inderal. Cardioversion if these methods are unsuccessful.
50.	Interpretation:	Wenckebach (Mobitz I).
	Treatment:	Oxygen, IV TKO, morphine for pain, watch for further slowing of the heart or more advanced heart block. If this occurs, may need to treat with atropine.

51. Interpretation: Complete heart block with a junctional escape rhythm.
    Treatment: Oxygen, IV TKO, atropine, Isuprel, transport for insertion of a pacemaker.
52. Interpretation: Ventricular standstill.
    Treatment: Assuming that CPR, Oxygen and the IV have all been started, administer sodium bicarbonate, Epinephrine, calcium chloride, and/or Isuprel.
53. Interpretation: Ventricular tachycardia going into an idioventricular rhythm.
    Treatment: Assist ventilations, CPR, IV TKO, sodium bicarbonate, Epinephrine or Isuprel. Prompt transport.
54. Interpretation: Sinus rhythm with first degree heart block with a depressed ST segment.
    Treatment: Oxygen, IV TKO, watch for further blocks or ventricular irritability, consider digitalis toxicity.
55. Interpretation: Wandering atrial pacemaker.
    Treatment: Oxygen, treat the knee injury.
56. Interpretation: Borderline sinus tachycardia with unifocal PVCs.
    Treatment: Low-flow oxygen, IV TKO, lidocaine bolus and drip if PVC's are not suppressed by oxygen.
57. Interpretation: Sinus tachycardia with multifocal and coupled PVCs.
    Treatment: Oxygen, IV TKO, lidocaine and Dopamine, Aramine, or Levophed; monitor closely.
58. Interpretation: Sinus rhythm with first degree heart block and intermittent second degree heart block /Wenckebach (Mobitz I).
    Treatment: Oxygen, IV TKO, morphine sulfate for pain. Watch closely for further block or drop in cardiac output. If this occurs, give atropine.
59. Interpretation: CHB with ventricular escape rhythm and underlying sinus tachycardia.
    Treatment: CPR, IV TKO, sodium bicarbonate, Isuprel and/or Epinephrine and calcium chloride.

60. Interpretation: Idioventricular rhythm, dying heart.
    Treatment: CPR, transport immediately; enroute start an IV of Ringer's Lactate and run it wide open, consider anti-shock trousers, administer sodium bicarbonate, Epinephrine, Isuprel, and/or calcium chloride.

PRACTICAL SKILLS

INTRODUCTION

This section will help you review the skills used in providing advanced care in the prehospital setting. As with the other parts of this book, the skills section assumes that you already know how to perform these techniques; therefore, it does not attempt to provide actual instruction.

A total of 25 commonly used skills have been selected and listed in alphabetical order. Each is summarized by a brief definition, along with indications, contraindications, and important points to remember when performing that skill. This short narrative is followed by Procedural Guidelines which list sequentially the steps that must be taken to complete that skill. This information can be easily adapted to conform to the local philosophies of your particular region.

Self-Assessment Exercises are included at the end of this section to allow you to test your academic knowledge of these skills. In order to develop competency in the skills areas, each exercise should be completed in conjunction with actual supervised performance of the skill.

To use this section, you should first modify the procedural guidelines to comply with the teachings in your own area. Review the information provided and perform each skill under the supervision of your instructor or someone from your base hospital. Then answer each of the self-assessment questions to ensure a total understanding of each skill.

Most of the skills included in this section were selected because they are used in many advanced life support (ALS) programs in the United States. Some of the skills included are less widely used, but are considered vital by one or more specific training programs. In an effort to provide a comprehensive resource for a wide variety of people, some procedures have been included that do not have documented field value. Therefore, it must be emphasized that inclusion of a skill in this section does not necessarily imply that the authors endorse its use in the prehospital setting.

Quite a few skills have been deliberately omitted from this review and may be noticed for their absence. All of the basic life support skills, e.g., cardiopulmonary resuscitation (CPR), bandaging, splinting, and control of bleeding were excluded because they are covered completely in texts at the basic level. Additionally, although extrication is considered extremely important for the ALS provider, this topic, too, has been thoroughly explained in other texts.

Several skills were omitted because they are impractical or they cause undue delay in the field, i.e., insertion of a urinary catheter and sophisticated auscultation techniques such as assessment of bowel sounds, fetal heart tones, and technical heart sounds.

Although most of the skills listed have fairly uniform performance criteria, some procedures must be modified according to the brand of product utilized in the performance of that skill. To facilitate explanation in these cases, specific brands were arbitrarily chosen for discussion. This does not imply an endorsement of that brand. To modify such descriptions to fit the product used in your area, refer to your lecture notes, your instructor, or the product literature.

ANTISHOCK TROUSERS (MAST III)

Although several antishock trousers have been developed with individual identifying features, most consist of a basic three-chambered inflatable garment designed to cover the lower extremities and the abdomen. When the trousers are applied to the patient in hypovolemic shock, they a) control bleeding by direct pressure, b) redirect available blood from the lower extremities to vital organs, and c) increase relative blood volume by about 1000 ml. They should be applied as soon as possible following the injury and used in conjunction with other standard shock measures.

The antishock trousers should be considered for any patient suspected of bleeding (internal or external) and who is exhibiting signs of shock such as diaphoresis, cold clammy skin, tachycardia and a drop in blood pressure. Although most commonly used for hemorrhage following trauma, the antishock trousers have also been used in other hypovolemic states, low resistance shock, and in cardiac arrests. Antishock trousers are contraindicated in the presence of isolated head injury, cardiopulmonary insufficiency, and major intrathoracic trauma or bleeding since the antishock trousers may aggravate these conditions. However in the presence of profound hypotension which does not respond to other measures, the antishock trousers may be necessary to sustain life in these patients.

The structure of the suit allows simultaneous or independent inflation of the three chambers. This flexibility allows the suit to be used in unusual circumstances such as pregnancy, bowel evisceration, presence of impaled objects, or marked abdominal distension.

Apply the suit so that its upper edge is just below the rib cage. Make sure all Velcro straps are secure and all valves are tightly closed before disconnecting the inflated suit from the pump.

During use, monitor the patient's vital signs closely to avoid IV fluid overload. Watch for signs of nausea and vomiting, or difficulty in breathing. If either of these occur, deflate the abdominal compartment slightly to help relieve the pressure. Do not remove the antishock trousers in the field, since to do so may throw the patient into sudden circulatory collapse and irreversible shock. Even in the hospital, the trousers should only be removed by a physician who is familiar with its use, and then only when all support services are ready.

PROCEDURAL GUIDELINES

Three-Chambered Antishock Trousers

1. Discuss indications for use of antishock trousers
2. Unfold garment completely and lay it flat on the ground or guerney
3. Attach foot pump and open stopcock valves
4. Place patient on the suit face up, so that the top of the garment is just below the lowest rib
5. Wrap each leg of the garment around patient's legs and secure with Velcro fasteners
6. Position abdominal section and secure it with the Velcro fastener
7. Use the foot pump to inflate trousers until air escapes through relief valves and/or patient's vital signs stabilize
8. Close all stopcock valves securely before disconnecting pump
9. Report to base hospital that application is complete and provide an update on patient's condition.

CARDIOVERSION

Cardioversion is the delivery of an electric shock to the heart by discharging a current directly to the chest wall. It differs from defibrillation in that the current is synchronized to be delivered on the QRS complex, thus avoiding discharge on the T wave. Cardioversion is used to convert uncompensated supraventricular or ventricular tachycardias. It is seldom used in the field to treat supraventricular tachycardias since other techniques such as vagal maneuvers or drugs are usually successful. Because ventricular tachycardia has a T wave, it should be cardioverted rather than defibrillated, if at all possible. Use caution when cardioverting a patient to whom digitalis has been administered.

Start an IV of D_5W and sedate the patient with Valium if he is not already unconscious. Transmit the EKG throughout the procedure and give continuous oxygen.

Before cardioverting, be sure that the synchronization button is on and flashing and/or that you can visualize the blip on the QRS complex. Select an initial watt/second (w/s) setting of 20–200 for cardioversion of supraventricular tachycardia. For ventricular tachycardia use 3.5–6 w/s per kg for patients up to 50 kg; over 50 kg, use full output of defibrillation. As with defibrillation, use adequate paddle pressure and apply the appropriate amount of gel or saline. All other safety precautions are the same as with defibrillation.

Following delivery of the countershock, assess the patient for improvement in vital signs, level of consciousness and rhythm. If necessary, repeat cardioversion at the same or increased w/s or resume other resuscitative measures such as CPR and drugs.

PROCEDURAL GUIDELINES

1. Identify the clinical indications for cardioversion in supraventricular and ventricular tachycardias
2. Sedate the patient (if alert)
3. Properly prepare paddles using gel, saline-soaked pads or commercial pads
4. Turn on defibrillator and select designated w/s setting
5. Press Synchronization button and check for synchronization blip on QRS complex
6. Press Charge button and wait for full charge
7. Demonstrate paddle placement
   a. right: right sternal border, 2nd intercostal space
   b. left: at apex
8. Apply paddles with approximately 15 pounds pressure
9. Emphasize safety precautions
   a. order "stand clear"
   b. disengage from physical contact with patient during discharge
   c. wipe excess gel, saline, or perspiration off patient
   d. keep hands off Discharge button until actually ready to initiate cardioversion
10. Simulate cardioversion on a special manikin or replace paddles in unit and discharge current
11. Check EKG and vital signs; report patient response

12. Discuss alternate anterior-posterior paddle placement and indications

CAROTID SINUS MASSAGE

Stimulation of the vagus nerve causes slowing of the sinus node and decreases conduction through the AV junction. Therefore, in supraventricular tachycardias, vagal stimulation is frequently an effective method of slowing or even converting these rhythms to a more adequate pattern. Any method of vagal stimulation should be performed in the prehospital setting only if the patient is not tolerating a supraventricular tachycardia and is experiencing signs and symptoms of decreased cardiac output.

There are two forms of vagal stimulation commonly used in the field, Valsalva's maneuver and carotid sinus massage. Both of these methods can be potentially lethal and must be ordered by the hospital. Prior to attempting any vagotonic maneuver, administer oxygen, start an IV of D$_5$W TKO and monitor the EKG. Have full resuscitative equipment ready and inform the patient of the procedure. Monitor vital signs before, during, and after the procedure.

Valsalva's maneuver is the most convenient of these mechanisms. It is performed by having the patient take a deep breath and bear down against his closed glottis, much like straining for a bowel movement. Although this appears to be a simple procedure, it can cause severe bradyarrhythmias including asystole, so monitor the EKG very closely. If Valsalva's maneuver doesn't convert the rhythm, carotid sinus massage may be necessary.

Carotid sinus massage is a noninvasive method of stimulating the vagus nerve. Because vagus nerve endings are located in the carotid sinus, external pressure to the neck at the site of the carotid sinus can cause the heart rate to decrease. Extreme caution must be used in performing this procedure as it can result in asystole. Prior to performing carotid sinus massage you must check for equality of carotid pulses and avoid massaging a side with a diminished pulse. Initially attempt to convert the rhythm by firm pressure alone. If this is ineffective, proceed to *cautiously* massage the carotid sinus. Massage only one side at a time, and discontinue massage at the first sign of a slowing in the rhythm. Do not massage for more than 5–10 seconds, and stop immediately if the patient shows signs of dizziness or other response.

When performing any vagotonic maneuver, transmit the EKG to the hospital throughout the procedure. Rhythms that may result from vagal stimulation include bradycardias, heart blocks, ventricular tachycardia, ventricular fibrillation, and asystole. Cerebral complications may include syncope, convulsions, or hemiplegia. Increased parasympathetic tone may produce hypotension, nausea, vomiting, or bronchospasm.

If vagal stimulation is unsuccessful in slowing or converting the rhythm, digoxin, Inderal or even cardioversion may be necessary.

Several other mechanisms, including the "diving seal" reflex and the orbital pressure maneuver, are also known to produce slowing of the heart rate. However, they have not been demonstrated to have an appropriate application in the prehospital setting, and have therefore been omitted from this discussion. It is also noted that vomiting has a vagotonic effect, and is often followed by a reflex bradycardia. However, induced vomiting may cause aspiration; therefore its use is not recommended.

PROCEDURAL GUIDELINES

1. Give indications for vagal stimulation
2. Ascertain that Valsalva's maneuver has been unsuccessful
3. Check to see that patient has oxygen and an IV, and is on a cardiac monitor
4. Explain the procedure to the patient
5. Prepare resuscitative equipment
6. Place patient in a supine position with head hyperextended; check for equality of carotid pulses, then rotate the head to expose appropriate carotid sinus
7. Properly locate carotid sinus at intersection of
   a. straight line down from ear to clavicle
   b. straight line back from larynx
8. Using the flat side of 2–3 fingers, press firmly over the carotid sinus.
9. If no response, massage the carotid sinus by pressing firmly toward cervical vertebrae and massaging up and back in a circular motion
10. Discontinue the procedure
    a. after 5–10 seconds, or
    b. at first sign of a slowing heart rate, or
    c. if patient experiences dizziness or altered level of consciousness

11. Repeat procedure once on opposite side if necessary and not contraindicated
12. Evaluate and report patient's response to treatment

CHEST AUSCULTATION

Chest auscultation is the act of listening to lung or heart sounds with a stethoscope. It is primarily used in the field to evaluate breath sounds and effectiveness of air exchange. Auscultation of lung sounds can detect rales, rhonchi, wheezes, or other unusual findings in patients with respiratory symptoms, chest pain, or unconsciousness. Auscultation techniques are also useful following trauma to detect absent or diminished breath sounds associated with pneumothorax or hemothorax.

Since lung sounds cannot be adequately auscultated through clothing, place the diaphragm of the stethoscope directly against the patient's skin. As the patient inhales and exhales, listen to air exchange while systematically moving the stethoscope across the chest wall until all lung fields have been auscultated. Lung sounds usually are best heard from the posterior thoracic cage. Report the type of lung sounds and where they were heard.

During transport, reevalute lung sounds, update vital signs, and report any changes in the patient's condition. This is especially important when medications such as Aminophylline or Lasix have been administered to alter the clinical condition.

Chest auscultation is also used to evaluate heart sounds. Muffled or distant heart sounds, along with increasing signs of shock following trauma, should suggest pericardial tamponade. You might need to determine heart rate by auscultation. This is particularly useful in the presence of pulse deficit, or when no peripheral pulse is palpable. Detailed differentiation of heart sounds such as S_3, S_4, and friction rubs is impractical for the field and should be reserved for hospital assessment.

PROCEDURAL GUIDELINES

1. Identify indications for auscultating the chest
2. Expose the patient's chest
3. Position patient
   a. have patient sit upright if he is alert
   b. if he is not alert, place patient first on his back, then on his side

4. Auscultate chest with diaphragm of stethoscope and check lung sounds
   a. instruct the patient to inhale and exhale through the mouth
   b. auscultate posterior and anterior lung fields in a systematic manner
   c. identify lung sounds detected
5. Place diaphragm of stethoscope over apex and auscultate heart sounds
   a. if respirations are noisy, instruct patient to hold his breath
   b. auscultate over apex of heart
   c. determine heart rate
   d. identify muffling, if present
6. Report findings

CRICOTHYROTOMY

Cricothyrotomy is the creation of an artificial airway in the trachea to bypass the site of an upper airway obstruction. It is a life-saving measure that should be performed *only* when all other methods of opening and maintaining a patent airway have failed.

The cricothyroid membrane is used because 1) it is easily located, 2) it can be quickly penetrated in an emergency situation, 3) it contains no vital structures, and 4) it is located below the vocal cords.

Bleeding is the most common complication of this procedure, but it is usually minor and controllable. Other complications include speech or nerve impairment (if the incision is made incorrectly), infection, or collapse of the cricoid cartilage itself. When performing this procedure, it is important to properly identify the landmarks and keep the incision small and in the midline.

Although the incision method provides greater air exchange, the puncture method is recommended because it is simpler and has a lesser potential for complications. To provide adequate air exchange, you may need to place additional cannulas adjacent to the first. After opening the airway, provide ventilatory assistance with high-flow oxygen. Following the procedure, transport promptly and monitor the patient closely.

PROCEDURAL GUIDELINES

Incision Method
1. Recognize indications for procedure
2. Select equipment

3. Place a small roll under patient's shoulders to slightly extend the neck
4. Locate cricothyroid membrane:
   a. properly locate the thyroid cartilage
   b. properly locate the cricoid cartilage
5. Prepare the skin with antiseptic swab and maintain aseptic technique
6. Stabilize thyroid cartilage between thumb and middle finger of one hand
7. Press index finger of same hand between the thyroid and cricoid cartilage to identify the cricothyroid membrane
8. Using index finger as a guide, make a small scalpel incision (2 cm) through the skin at the midline
9. Make second incision through the cricothyroid membrane, taking care not to incise laterally or too deeply
10. Rotate knife handle 90° to widen opening
11. Insert a cannula, tubing, or penshaft to maintain an airway
12. Check placement of the airway by
    a. ventilating (as necessary) and watching the chest rise
    b. listening for air exchange at the site
    c. observing patient for color and respiratory improvement
13. Secure airway with tape
14. Administer high-flow oxygen and continue ventilatory assistance as needed
15. Update patient status to base hospital and transport immediately

PROCEDURAL GUIDELINES

Puncture Method
1. Recognize indications for procedure
2. Select equipment
3. Place a small roll under patient's shoulders to slightly extend neck
4. Locate cricothyroid membrane:
   a. properly locate thyroid cartilage
   b. properly locate cricoid cartilage
5. Prepare the skin with antiseptic swab and maintain aseptic technique

6. Stabilize thyroid cartilage between thumb and middle finger of one hand
7. Press index finger of same hand between the thyroid and cricoid cartilage to identify cricothyroid membrane
8. Using index finger as a guide
   a. rest middle or ring finger of hand holding needle/cannula on the skin to stabilize and prevent needle from penetrating membrane too deeply
   b. make a puncture in the midline with a thrusting motion
   c. insert cannula at a 90° angle
9. After entry into trachea, remove needle, holding cannula in place.
10. Check placement of airway by
    a. ventilating (as necessary) and watching chest rise
    b. listening for air exchange at the site
    c. observing patient for color and respiratory improvement
11. Advance cannula into trachea at a 45° angle
12. Tape the cannula securely in place
13. Administer high-flow oxygen or ventilatory assistance as needed
14. Place additional needles/cannulas if needed, to assure adequate air exchange
15. Provide update of patient's status to base hospital and transport immediately.

DEFIBRILLATION

Defibrillation is the application of a direct electrical current to the chest wall of a patient in cardiac arrest. The purpose of this procedure is to convert non-viable rhythms such as ventricular fibrillation or ventricular tachycardia to a more life-sustaining pattern. Although electrical countershock is not the treatment of choice for a patient in asystole, it is sometimes tried as a last resort.

Do not defibrillate until you have looked at the patient and felt for the pulse, since a loose lead wire or patient movement may mimic ventricular fibrillation. The ability to take a "quick look" through the defibrillator paddles enables you to identify the rhythm in less time than it takes to charge the paddles, thereby making blind defibrillation inappropriate.

Select a watt/second setting of 3.5—6 w/s per kilogram for patients up to 50 kg. For patients over 50 kg, use full output of the defibrillator.

Because the defibrillator delivers a large electrical current, the safety of all personnel involved is as important as the safety of the patient. Defibrillation should be avoided if the patient is very wet or is lying in a puddle of water, as this will disperse the current and endanger both the patient and the paramedic. Burns and arcing of current can be prevented or reduced by using appropriate amounts of saline or gel and firm pressure on the patient's chest. Check to see that everyone is clear of the patient before discharging the current. Personnel providing ventilation and chest compression should continue until the actual time of discharge, when they should pull away momentarily. The person holding the IV line must stand clear of the patient, but will not need to break contact with the IV as the current is not conducted through the line. Because defibrillation induces a seizure of skeletal muscles, the extremity with the IV should be immobilized carefully to prevent dislodgement of the IV line. If you don't see a generalized seizure at the time of defibrillation, you should suspect that the current was inadequate.

When defibrillating children, use special pediatric paddles. If pediatric paddles are not available, the anterior-posterior paddle position is most appropriate. This alternate paddle position is also useful when defibrillating obese or barrel-chested patients, or when normal paddle placement is hampered, as by an internal pacemaker.

Immediately following defibrillation resume CPR and reassess the patient. Response to defibrillation is best evaluated by palpating central pulses and looking for a conversion of the EKG rhythm. Defibrillation most commonly converts ventricular fibrillation into bradycardias, including idioventricular rhythm and supraventricular bradycardias. These rhythms can often be improved by using drugs.

Patients in arrest from ventricular fibrillation are assumed to be in concurrent respiratory acidosis. Correction of the acidotic state will improve the potential for conversion of the ventricular rhythm. For this reason, sodium bicarbonate should be given prior to defibrillation in an unwitnessed arrest. Epinephrine may also be administered as a means of improving chances of conversion. Lidocaine is likely to reduce the ventricular irritability; therefore it is indicated during or after the arrest situation to prevent return to ventricular fibrillation.

As with all portable emergency equipment, the defibrillator must always be kept in operational condition. This requires you to check equipment daily to be sure that the battery level is adequate, that all parts are available and functioning, and that the equipment performs as it should.

PROCEDURAL GUIDELINES	1. Recognize clinical indications for defibrillation
	2. Properly prepare paddles using
	  a. gel
	  b. saline-soaked pads
	  c. commercial pads
	3. Turn defibrillator on and select proper w/s setting
	4. Press Charge button and wait for unit to reach full charge
	5. Demonstrate paddle placement
	  a. right: right sternal border, 2nd intercostal space
	  b. left: at the apex
	6. Apply paddles with approximately 15 lbs pressure
	7. Emphasize safety precautions:
	  a. order "stand clear"
	  b. discontinue physical contact with the patient during discharge
	  c. wipe excess gel or saline from the patient
	  d. keep hands off Discharge button until actual defibrillation
	8. Simulate defibrillation on a special manikin, or replace paddles in unit and discharge current
	9. Check pulses and EKG; order "resume CPR" as needed
	10. Discuss alternate anterior-posterior paddle placement and indications

EKG MONITORING AND TELEMETRY

Electrocardiographic monitoring is the graphic display of the electrical activity of the heart. It is of vital importance in delivering effective prehospital management of problems that influence cardiac activity. EKG monitoring should be a priority for those patients with chest pain, difficult breathing, irregular pulse, unconsciousness or profound shock. Monitoring is also done whenever any medication is given that may influence heart rate and rhythm. Monitor the EKG in all questionable situations as a precautionary measure to augment patient assessment.

Remember that good lead contact is essential. You may need to apply extra gel, dry the diaphoretic patient, shave excess hair or abrade the skin to obtain a good EKG complex. Know how to troubleshoot equipment to alleviate artifact and 60-cycle interference. When faced with a straight line or what appears to be ventricular fibrillation, check both the patient and the connections to rule out a mechanical problem such as a loose lead wire. When connecting the cables, assure that lead wires are attached to the corresponding electrodes or the EKG readout will be inaccurate. Both Lead II and MCl_1 are good monitoring leads because they follow the conduction pathways of the heart and therefore show well defined P waves. This allows for easier detection of arrhythmias.

Place the monitor where it is most visible, keep a close watch on the rhythm to detect any abnormalities and anticipate the types of arrhythmias that may occur. Most patients who require EKG monitoring will also require oxygen, IV TKO, and possibly antiarrhythmic medications. Telemetry during cardiac arrest may be done periodically or sometimes even constantly to keep the hospital informed of the situation. When sending the EKG via telemetry remember to a) begin with a calibration signal, b) switch your radio mode to EKG and c) allow sufficient time for the hospital to evaluate the rhythm. Avoid interjecting unnecessary voice communications during the EKG transmission as this will distort the cardiac pattern.

PROCEDURAL GUIDELINES

Monitoring

1. Insert lead wires into corresponding patient cable connections
2. Attach chest electrodes
   a. prepare skin
   b. connect lead wires to electrode pads
   c. apply electrodes in correct position on chest wall
3. Attach patient cable to oscilloscope
4. Turn on oscillosope
5. Select appropriate lead for optimal rhythm interpretation
6. Adjust speed and/or gain if needed
7. Interpret arrhythmias displayed on screen
8. Report rhythm interpretation to base hospital and request confirmation

9. If monitor has graphic readout, produce a legible rhythm strip
10. Recognize and correct
    - 60-cycle interference
    - loose electrode or wire
    - artifact
    - muscle tremors, patient movement

PROCEDURAL GUIDELINES

Telemetry
1. Attach oscilloscope to radio via connecting cable
2. Switch dial on radio from *Voice* to *EKG*
3. Send brief calibration signal to hospital
4. Allow sufficient time for EKG transmission to hospital
5. Identify rhythm and request verification
6. Identify and correct equipment problems as they arise

ENDOTRACHEAL INTUBATION

Endotracheal (ET) intubation is the insertion of a tube directly into the trachea to open the airway and provide a pathway for ventilatory assistance. An ET tube is indicated in the field when a patient is not breathing effectively, or is not breathing at all. Intubation is contraindicated in upper airway obstruction due to foreign bodies. It should be used with caution in laryngeal edema or in patients with mandibular or cervical fractures, since attempts at intubation may aggravate these conditions.

The major field complication is due to improper placement into the esophagus which in effect forms a total airway obstruction and will result in death if not recognized and corrected. Other immediate complications include aspiration, trauma and/or perforation of the esophagus or pharynx, insertion into the right mainstem bronchus resulting in a left pneumothorax, bronchospasm, laryngospasm, hypoxemia, cardiac arrhythmias, and irritation of the carina with subsequent coughing.

Before inserting the airway, position the patient for maximum visual advantage and have suction available. Ventilate with 100% oxygen prior to and following intubation. Have all equipment ready and functioning. Avoid pronounced hyperextension of the neck and never insert the ET tube without direct visualization of the vocal cords. Keep the laryngoscope off the teeth to prevent chipping, which

367

could result in aspiration of tooth fragments by the patient. Once the tube is inserted, inflate the cuff and make sure it is properly positioned by auscultating both lungs for adequate breath sounds. Secure the tube in place with adhesive tape.

PROCEDURAL GUIDELINES

1. Establish need for intubation, i.e., respiratory arrest or inadequate ventilatory exchange
2. Assures that EKG is being monitored
3. Select proper equipment and assure proper functioning
4. Select the appropriate ET tube and lubricate with water-soluble lubricant
5. Have suction and oxygen prepared and available
6. Position patient's head so that trachea and oropharynx are aligned:
   a. place patient in supine position
   b. approach patient's head from above
   c. place pillow or blanket under neck or shoulders
   d. extend head by moving the chin up and back ("sniffing" position)
7. Ventilate with 100% oxygen
8. Grip handle of laryngoscope with left hand so that knuckles are parallel with the blade
9. Insert blade of laryngoscope along the right side of the tongue to its base, and displaces the tongue to the left
   a. advance the curved blade to the base of the tongue at the epiglottis, or
   b. advance the straight blade until the tip is under the epiglottis
10. Lift laryngoscope slightly upward and forward with the left hand to extend jaw further:
    a. lift with the shoulder, keeping wrist straight and firm
    b. avoid pressing laryngoscope against patient's teeth
11. Visualize vocal cords
12. Using the right hand, insert the endotracheal tube with its curve facing forward until cuff passes vocal cords

13. Remove the laryngoscope carefully
14. Assure proper placement:
    a. ventilate while auscultating for bilateral lung sounds
    b. watch for chest to rise
15. While ventilating patient, inflate cuff until expired air no longer leaks around cuff, then add 0.5–1 ml more air to assure seal
16. Ventilate with 100% oxygen
17. Insert oropharyngeal airway to act as bite block
18. Securely tape tube in place
19. Continue ventilatory efforts, suctioning as necessary

ESOPHAGEAL OBTURATOR AIRWAY

The esophageal obturator airway (EOA) is a cuffed tube which seals off the esophagus and channels ventilated air into the trachea. The concurrent use of a nasogastric (NG) tube either passed through or around the EOA, allows decompression of the stomach and prevents regurgitation. Because the EOA seals off the stomach from the airway, its use during CPR has greatly reduced the incidence of aspiration as a complication.

The EOA is indicated in an unconscious, apneic adult. It can be placed blindly without the need to see the oral anatomy and can be inserted with the patient's head in a neutral or slightly flexed position. It is contraindicated in any patient who is conscious and/or breathing effectively because the gag reflex may still be present, and emesis with aspiration may result at the time of insertion. The EOA should not be inserted in a patient with suspected narcotic overdose to whom Narcan will be administered, because the patient is expected to regain consciousness rapidly. It should be used with caution in severe facial trauma or known esophageal disease. Unfortunately, the EOA cannot be used on children because it is not yet available in pediatric sizes.

Before inflating the balloon, assure correct placement by giving one quick breath through the tube and watching for the chest to rise. Auscultate the chest during ventilation to evaluate adequacy of expansion. Remove the tube at once if you suspect placement in the trachea. Make sure you have an airtight seal around the mask, and pull the jaw forward for normal airway management. The EOA should not be removed in the field unless the patient actively resists it.

Do not remove it without suctioning and positioning the patient to avoid aspiration.

The most common complication of this procedure is improper removal by personnel who are unfamiliar with its use. To avoid this, make sure all Emergency Department and support personnel are aware of the function and position of the EOA. Endotracheal intubation may be performed with the EOA in place.

PROCEDURAL GUIDELINES

1. Select equipment and assure proper functioning
2. Lubricate tube and attach mask
3. Properly position head in neutral or flexed position
4. Insert tube until mask rests on face (displace tongue laterally and follow curvature of oropharynx)
5. Check for placement:
   a. make airtight seal with mask
   b. immediately give one large breath through tube and watch for chest to rise
   c. if chest does not rise, pull tube out, ventilate and attempt again
   d. if chest expands, inflate cuff with 35 ml air
6. Ventilate patient with supplemental oxygen
   a. maintain airtight seal with mask to face
   b. auscultate chest bilaterally
   c. watch for chest movement
7. Suction oropharynx as needed
8. Pass NG tube as ordered around or through the tube
9. Remove EOA when appropriate
   a. turn patient to side
   b. deflate cuff
   c. use suction as needed
   d. gently remove tube
   e. continue supplemental oxygen

INTRACARDIAC INJECTIONS

An intracardiac (IC) injection deposits medication directly into the ventricular chamber of the heart. It is usually performed during cardiac arrest when a standard IV route is unobtainable, or when a direct pharmacological effect on the myocardium is desired. The medications most commonly given as IC injections in the field are Epinephrine and calcium chloride.

Because of the severity of complications associated with IC injections, there is significant controversy over its use. When used as a final resuscitative effort, however, its potential benefits outweigh the possible side effects.

Some degree of myocardial damage probably occurs with every IC injection. Most damage occurs when the heart is still fibrillating or when the needle is jarred during the procedure. The needle tip may tear a coronary artery, the myocardium, or the pericardium. When there is bleeding within the pericardial sac, a pericardial tamponade may develop. Other complications which may be caused by IC injections are hemothorax and pneumothorax, neither of which is a priority during an arrest situation.

When performing an IC injection, do not interrupt CPR any longer than necessary. In order to keep the interruption minimal, locate the landmarks for the injection and prepare the medication while CPR is still in progress. Aspirate continuously while advancing the needle through the myocardium. When a free flow of blood appears, inject the medication quickly. Immediately after withdrawing the needle, resume CPR to circulate the drug. Assess the effectiveness of the drug by palpating the pulses and observing the EKG monitor.

Although indications for an IC injection in a child are the same as for an adult, the different anatomical position of the heart in infants and children requires variances in technique. These variances are included in the procedural guidelines.

PROCEDURAL GUIDELINES

1. Identify indications for IC injections.
2. Prepare the medication, using aseptic technique
   a. select a preloaded syringe, or
   b. withdraw the medication from an ampule
3. Recheck drugs, dosage, and route
4. Locate injection site and prepare the skin
5. Maintaining aseptic technique, insert needle through the skin with a quick thrust
   a. 4th intercostal space, 2 cm left of sternum at a 90° angle
   b. 5th intercostal space, 2 cm left of ster-

      num; aim toward head at a 70°-80°
      angle

  c. subxiphoid, immediately below and left
      of xiphoid process; aim toward left
      shoulder at a 45° angle

6. Advance needle slowly while aspirating
7. When blood flows freely into syringe, quickly inject drug into ventricular cavity
8. Quickly withdraw needle, pressing alcohol swab or gauze over site
9. Direct others to resume CPR
10. Assess effectiveness of medication by evaluating pulse and EKG
11. Report to hospital that drug is "on board" and give patient response
12. Record administration of drug and patient response
13. Demonstrate variations for infants and small children

- infants (newborn to 3 years)
  a. use subxiphoid site only
  b. use 1½-inch 21-gauge needle
  c. insert needle at 20° angle, aiming toward left midclavicular line
- young children (3–12 years)
  a. use 3-inch, 20-gauge needle
  b. subxiphoid or third or fourth intercostal spaces are the only acceptable sites
  c. insert needle
    - subxiphoid, 20° angle, aim for third intercostal space, midclavicular line
    - third intercostal space, 90° angle, straight in
    - fourth intercostal space, aim for head at a 70–80° angle

INTRAMUSCULAR AND SUBCUTANEOUS INJECTIONS

Medications may be injected directly into the patient's tissues either intramuscularly (IM) or subcutaneously (SC). These routes are used when an IV cannot be established, or when a slower absorption rate is preferred over the IV route. Both methods are contraindicated in profound shock states because peripheral circulation is impaired and the drug will remain unabsorbed in the tissues. Complications include nerve damage and local infection, both of which are associated with improper technique.

IM injections are usually given in the deltoid muscle, but may be given into any major muscle mass. Choose a 21-gauge needle, 1–1½ inches long, and insert the needle at a 90° angle to deposit the drug into the muscle layer. Medications commonly given by the IM route include Benadryl, Valium, atropine sulfate and morphine sulfate.

Subcutaneous injections are given at a 45° angle into the fatty tissues of the upper arm, abdomen or thigh. They require a smaller needle, usually 23-gauge, ⅝-inch. The SC route is used to administer Epinephrine 1:1000 when treating asthma or anaphylaxis, or morphine sulfate.

Before giving any drug, make sure the order includes the route as well as the dosage. Explain the procedure to the patient and ask about allergies. Using aseptic technique, insert the needle quickly, aspirate, inject the drug, and withdraw the needle smoothly. Following the injection, evaluate the patient carefully for both desired and untoward effects. Depending on the properties of the drug and the patient's status, these effects may be delayed for 5–10 minutes.

PROCEDURAL GUIDELINES

Intramuscular (IM) and Subcutaneous (SC) Injections

1. Prepare patient by explaining procedure, checking for allergies, and positioning patient as needed
2. Gather equipment
3. Prepare needle and syringe, maintaining aseptic technique throughout the procedure
4. Withdraw medication from
   a. ampul
   b. vial
      - swab top of vial
      - inject proportional volume of air into bottle and aspirate correct dosage
5. Check for and displace air bubbles prior to injection
6. Select appropriate site
7. Prep skin with antiseptic swab
8. Recheck medication and dosage
9. Properly support skin

10. Insert needle with bevel up
    - IM injections, needle should be at a 90° angle
    - SC injections, needle should be at a 45° angle
11. Release skin before injecting solution
12. Aspirate to ensure needle is not in a blood vessel
13. Inject solution slowly and smoothly
14. Support skin with antiseptic swab while quickly withdrawing needle
15. Massage skin to help with absorption of drug
16. Report that drug is "on board"
17. Monitor and report patient's response to drug
18. Chart medication on prehospital report form

IV INSERTION INTO THE EXTERNAL JUGULAR VEIN

An IV catheter may be inserted into the external jugular vein in order to infuse various medications and IV solutions into the circulatory system. This route is selected only after other peripheral IV attempts have been unsuccessful and an IV line is essential to patient management.

The external jugular vein is a large peripheral vessel which runs superficially along the side of the neck between the ear and the midclavicular line. It can be distended by a) tamponading (compressing) the vein immediately above the clavicle, b) lowering the head, and/or c) elevating the lower extremities if the patient is in severe circulatory collapse.

Complications which may occur from external jugular cannulation include air embolism, pneumothorax, hematoma and infiltration. Air embolus can be avoided by placing the patient in a Trendelenberg position, clearing the IV tubing of air, and firmly tamponading the vein while connecting the tubing to the cannula. To help prevent pneumothorax, puncture the vein as closely as possible to the angle of the jaw. Watch closely for signs of hematoma formation or infiltration. If either occurs, discontinue the IV and apply firm pressure.

Following the procedure, auscultate the lungs frequently to detect the occurrence of pneumothorax or fluid overload. Tape the cannula securely to avoid possible dislodgement caused by patient movement.

PROCEDURAL GUIDELINES

1. Gather equipment
2. Place patient in supine position, with head lowered slightly and turned at a 45°–60° angle from the midline
3. Locate external jugular vein
4. Cleanse skin thoroughly with antiseptic swabs
5. Stabilize the skin above proposed puncture site by using gentle countertraction
6. Distend vein by
   a. tamponading just above clavicle
   b. lowering patient's head
   c. elevating lower extremities
7. Using aseptic technique, make venipuncture midway between the angle of the jaw and the midclavicular line.
8. Make first thrust lateral to vein to penetrate the skin
9. Once through the skin, adjust angle and cannulate vein itself, while aspirating for blood return
10. When vein has been penetrated, remove needle and advance cannula
11. After cannula is inserted, tamponade vein at end of catheter.
12. Draw blood if ordered, maintaining compression on vein while removing the syringe
13. Connect IV tubing *securely* to cannula end and release tamponade
14. Set IV flow rate as ordered and adjust as needed
15. Tape needle (or catheter) and tubing securely in place
16. Check IV site frequently
17. Auscultate lung sounds to rule out pneumothorax and fluid overload
18. Report completed cannulation to base hospital

19. Explain variations for infants and children
    a. have assistant support child's head and neck over edge of table while securing shoulders firmly on table
    b. mummy-wrap wriggling infants if necessary
    c. if child is awake, induce venous distention by stimulating his cry

IV INSERTION INTO PERIPHERAL VEIN

The insertion of an indwelling catheter into a vein is done to establish direct access into the circulatory system. This line can then be used to administer specific medications or replace intravenous fluids. The vein is often just kept open in case medications are needed.

The site for an IV varies according to the patient's veins and clinical condition. Ideally, the most distal veins of the upper extremities should be used first so that other veins are availabe if repeated cannulations are necessary. In life-threatening emergencies, the larger veins of the antecubital fossa can be used because of their easy access.

To facilitate venous distension, apply a constriction band, lower the extremity, or stroke the vein upward. With difficult veins, the application of heat or an ace wrap may further distend the vein. You may have to omit the tourniquet if the patient is extremely hypertensive or has fragile veins.

To stabilize the vein during the puncture, insert the needle at a bifurcation or apply countertraction and anchor the vein with your fingers. Secure the cannula or needle but avoid taping around the entire extremity as this may create a tourniquet effect if infiltration occurs. Use an arm board whenever the IV has been started near a joint.

If the IV begins to flow poorly or there is redness, pain, or swelling around the IV site, suspect infiltration and restart the IV as needed. Throughout the procedure, use aseptic technique to reduce the occurrence of local and systemic infections. To prevent air embolism, clear the tubing of air initially and assure that all connections are tightly secured.

Closely watch the IV drip rate, especially after giving an IV medication or changing the patient's position. Auscultate lung sounds frequently and reduce the IV flow if pulmonary congestion develops.

PROCEDURAL GUIDELINES

1. Gather and prepare equipment
2. Apply a constricting band and assess peripheral pulse
3. Identify an appropriate vein
4. If necessary, produce additional venous distension by one or more of the following:
   a. tapping the vein
   b. stroking the vein upward
   c. lowering the extremity
5. Prep site with antiseptic swab; maintain aseptic technique throughout procedure
6. Stabilize vein
   a. use fingers to apply countertraction
   b. insert needle at bifurcation when possible
7. Puncture vein with
   • cannula over needle
   a. pierce skin at a 20° angle on top of or along side the vein
   b. adjust angle of insertion to enter vein
   c. watch or aspirate for flashback of blood
   d. advance cannula and remove needle
   • scalp vein needle
   a. pierce skin at a 20° angle on top of or along side the vein
   b. adjust angle of insertion to enter vein
   c. watch or aspirate for flashback of blood
   d. advance needle into vein
8. Tamponade above the puncture site to reduce bleeding
9. Connect IV tubing firmly to cannula/scalp vein
10. Release constricting band
11. Start IV flow and check for infiltration
12. Secure IV by
    a. applying tape
    b. applying armboard as needed
13. Recheck IV flow rate, and adjust as needed
14. Evaluate patient's lung sounds and respiratory rate
15. Report IV initiation
16. Reassess IV for patency and drip rate

IV INSERTION INTO THE SUBCLAVIAN VEIN

A catheter may be inserted into the subclavian vein to provide access for IV fluids and/or medications. The subclavian site for IV initiation has the following advantages over peripheral sites: 1) it is a large central vein; 2) it provides for quick absorption of medications; 3) it handles a large volume of fluid easily, and 4) it allows for easy insertion of a transvenous pacemaker wire if needed. This site is used when a peripheral line is not possible or in cardiac arrest situations.

This procedure can produce severe complications such as hemothorax, pneumothorax, and lacerated veins or arteries. To help prevent pneumothorax, instruct the alert patient to take shallow breaths during the procedure. In addition, avoid inserting the needle too deeply, or entering the vein at the wrong angle, or changing the angle of the needle carelessly.

Another major complication is air embolism. There are four ways to help prevent this complication: 1) place the patient in Trendelenberg position; 2) tamponade the catheter following removal of the needle; 3) keep all IV line connections secure, and 4) assure that all air is removed from the IV line.

Prepare the skin well to reduce the incidence of infection. Once the cannula is in place, tape it securely and prevent excessive patient movement. If there is too much torsion on the IV cannula, it can be displaced, causing severe bleeding into the thorax. Lung sounds should be auscultated following the procedure to rule out a pneumothorax. If this is suspected, transport the patient promptly.

Following correct placement, adjust the IV rate and monitor the patient closely for possible fluid overload since the subclavian vein is very large and can accommodate a large volume of fluid very rapidly.

PROCEDURAL GUIDELINES

1. Gather equipment
2. Prepare patient and explain procedure (if conscious)
3. Position patient
   a. supine
   b. Trendelenberg
   c. turn head to opposite side of puncture
   d. place pillow under shoulders (optional)
4. Prepare area with antiseptic swab (midsternum lateral to shoulder joint, including suprasternal notch)

5. Instruct alert patient to take shallow breaths
6. Insert cannula, using aseptic technique 1 cm below the midclavicular point at $10°-15°$ angle to skin
7. Advance cannula slowly toward upper border of suprasternal notch
8. Assess entrance into vein by observing a free flow of blood into cannula
9. Advance cannula to thread it into vein
10. Tamponade end of cannula, quickly pull out needle and connect IV tubing to cannula
11. Tape cannula securely in place and apply dressing
12. Establish drip rate
13. Auscultate chest, and observe for complications
14. Record and report completion of procedure

IV MEDICATION
ADMINISTRATION

Medications administered intravenously are injected directly into the vascular system. The intravenous (IV) route is preferred when an immediate response is needed in such life threatening situations as cardiac and/or respiratory arrest, or when peripheral circulation is impaired, as with myocardial infarction, acute respiratory emergencies, shock, and drug overdose. While most IV medications are injected via an indwelling IV line, they may also be given directly into a vein or infused gradually after being diluted in a Volutrol or in a bag of IV solution. The method of administration will vary according to the properties of the specific medication and the desired effect on an individual patient.

Before injecting any IV medication, ensure that infiltration has not occurred. Infiltration will impede absorption, and in some instances may cause tissue necrosis.

Since the IV route provides rapid distribution of the medication, therapeutic actions as well as side effects will occur very quickly. Therefore, it is essential to monitor the patient's response closely. Before administering any drug, check the patient's history for drug allergies and make sure the drug is not outdated. Always verify drug orders with the base hospital, prepare and administer doses accurately, report responses promptly, and record all drug administrations on the patient's record. Question any order which appears inappropriate, and withhold administration of the drug if the question cannot be resolved.

PROCEDURAL GUIDELINES

Direct IV Push

1. Question patient regarding allergies
2. Identify medication to be given by name, dosage, and route
3. Prepare prescribed medication by assembling a preloaded syringe, or drawing the appropriate dose from an ampule or vial
4. Apply a tourniquet and select a vein
5. Prepare puncture site with antiseptic swab; maintain aseptic technique throughout procedure
6. After rechecking medication and dosage, insert needle at a 10° angle to the skin and advance into vein
7. Aspirate for blood return
8. Remove tourniquet
9. Inject medication at appropriate rate, aspirating at intervals to ensure that needle remains in vein
10. Remove needle and compress site to prevent formation of a hematoma
11. Report to base hospital that drug is "on board"
12. Monitor and report patient's response to drug
13. Chart medication on prehospital report form

PROCEDURAL GUIDELINES

IV Push via IV Line

1. Question patient regarding allergies
2. Identify medication to be given by name, dosage, and route
3. Prepare prescribed medication by assembling a preloaded syringe, or drawing appropriate dose from an ampule or vial
4. Select injection site closest to patient and wipe with antiseptic swab

5. Recheck medication and dosage; administer through IV injection site, maintaining aseptic technique
   a. pinch off IV flow above injection site
   b. inject at proper rate for that drug
   c. reestablishes flow
   d. flush IV line
   e. readjust drip rate as needed
6. Report to base hospital that drug is "on board"
7. Monitor and report patient's response to drug
8. Chart medication on prehospital report form

PROCEDURAL GUIDELINES

IV Volutrol
1. Question patient regarding allergies
2. Identify medication to be given by name, dosage, and route
3. Set up an IV bag using a Volutrol administration set
   a. fill Volutrol with desired amount of solution
   b. run solution through drip chamber and tubing
   c. close valve between IV bag and Volutrol
   d. open air valve
4. Add medication to Volutrol
   a. wipe injection site with antiseptic swab
   b. recheck medication and dosage and inject drug through injection site on Volutrol
   c. label Volutrol with medication, dosage and time
5. Piggyback this IV set into main IV line and secure with tape; close main IV
6. Regulate drip rate by adjusting flow-regulation valve below Volutrol
7. Report medication drip in progress
8. Observe patient's vital signs and report changes
9. When volume has been infused, report drug is "on board"

10. Shut off flow on Volutrol tubing and reestablish IV flow on main IV line
11. Record drug administration and patient response on prehospital report form

PROCEDURAL GUIDELINES

IV Drip

1. Question patient regarding allergies
2. Identify medication to be given by name, dosage and route
3. Set up a new IV bag, with tubing
4. Wipe injection site on bag with antiseptic swab
5. Recheck medication and dosage and inject it into IV bag while maintaining aseptic technique
6. Label bag with medication, dosage, date and time
7. Squeeze or tilt bag to mix medication; fill tubing
8. Piggyback this IV into main IV line and secure it in place with tape; close off main IV
9. Adjust flow to specified rate, or titrate to pulse or blood pressure
10. Assess patient's vital signs (including lung sounds) frequently
11. Report to base hospital
    a. IV solution in progress
    b. rate of infusion
    c. patient's response to medication
12. Record drug information and patient response on prehospital report form

IV SET-UP

The selection and preparation of IV equipment is essential prior to cannulation of the vein. To save time when initiating an IV, use another member of your team to prepare the set-up while you select the insertion site. Specify which equipment you need assembled.

The size and type of IV needle you select will vary with the size of the patient's veins, the clinical indication for the IV, and to a small degree, your individual preference. Use large-bore cannulas in hypovolemic conditions when fluid replacement is needed. The smaller scalp vein needles can be used for children, elderly patients with fragile veins and TKO IVs. Cannulas are generally preferred over scalp-vein needles because they are less likely to infiltrate.

Select the IV administration set depending upon the desired rate of infusion. The standard maxidrip set administers one ml in 10–15 drops and is used for volume replacement. The pedidrip set delivers one ml in 60 drops and is safer to use whenever a controlled infusion rate is required. Add extension tubing to the IV administration set as needed.

A Volutrol or similar volume control chamber is an important measure in managing very young, old, or critically ill patients who could not tolerate a large volume of fluids. It is also necessary for diluting certain drugs used in the field. The Volutrol may come as a part of the IV administration set (usually with a pedidrip) or it may be added to the set-up between the bag and the tubing.

Before administering an IV, check each solution container for leaks, obvious contamination, and expiration date. The Viaflex bags have several advantages over bottles, as they can be manually compressed to increase the IV flow rate and are unbreakable. However, caution must be used to prevent puncturing the bag. The manufacturer warns that marking with a felt pen directly on the bag can contaminate the solution, so use an adhesive label instead.

PROCEDURAL GUIDELINES

1. Gather equipment and select appropriate IV administration set
2. Maintain aseptic technique throughout procedure
3. Remove IV solution bag from outer wrapping
   a. check expiration date
   b. check bag for leakage or cloudy solution
   c. remove tab from port for IV tubing insertion
4. Prepare the IV set by closing drip regulator below drip chamber, and uncapping spiked end of IV tubing
5. Firmly insert spike of IV administration set into port of IV bag and pierce diaphragm
6. Fill IV tubing with fluid
   a. squeeze drip chamber to fill it no more than half way

      b. open drip regulator to allow fluid to fill rest of the tubing

      c. uncap distal end of tubing to evacuate air from tubing as necessary

      d. recap tubing to maintain sterility

7. Ensure that all air has been evacuated from tubing

8. Insert IV extension tubing and/or stopcock at distal end of IV administration set and flush with IV fluid.

MAGILL FORCEPS

The Magill forceps and laryngoscope are instruments used for removing an object obstructing the upper airway. This procedure intervenes in a life-threatening emergency; therefore, you must perform it rapidly and without delay. The laryngoscope provides illumination of the posterior oropharynx, which allows you to view the obstruction. The Magill forceps are then used to grasp and remove the foreign matter. Use this procedure only on an *unconscious* patient and in conjunction with other maneuvers for airway obstruction, i.e., back blows and manual thrusts.

Complications include laryngospasm, soft tissue damage, and chipped teeth. Avoid these complications by exercising caution when inserting and removing these instruments. Particularly avoid resting the laryngoscope blade on the teeth. Check the laryngoscope daily to ensure that the battery and bulb are operational.

Manage the patient with high flow oxygen, cardiac monitoring and suctioning as needed.

PROCEDURAL GUIDELINES

1. Approach supine patient's head from above.

2. Hyperextend patient's head and neck unless contraindicated

3. Insert a bite stick, if feasible

4. Insert laryngoscope

      a. grasp handle with left hand, so that knuckles are parallel to blade

      b. place blade of laryngoscope to the right of tongue and displace tongue to left

      c. pull slightly up and out in direction of handle, extending jaw further

5. Visualize foreign object
6. Hold Magill forceps in right hand, palm down, with closed tips curving down
7. Insert closed tips of forceps down to object; be careful not to push the object further down into the airway
8. Open tips and clamp them firmly around object (If object cannot be grasped with tips of forceps, deflect object to one side to open airway)
9. Remove object by carefully pulling forceps out
10. Remove laryngoscope carefully (reverse insertion procedure)
11. When object has been removed (or displaced to one side), continue with airway management.

NASOGASTRIC INTUBATION

A nasogastric (NG) tube is inserted into the stomach via the nose to relieve distension caused by foods, fluids, blood or air. If left uncorrected, the increased intraabdominal pressure can cause vomiting and subsequent aspiration, bradycardia, or decreased lung expansion. This procedure is used in the treatment of near drowning, cardiac arrest, upper GI hemorrhage, drug overdose and poisonings.

Lubricate the NG tube generously to facilitate passage. Place the patient in high Fowler's position and advance the tube while he swallows or sips small amounts of water. If the patient doesn't swallow, gently stroke downward on his throat to stimulate the swallowing reflex. Monitor the patient closely while inserting the NG tube since vagal stimulation may induce arrhythmias.

Once the tube has been inserted, verify proper placement by aspirating for stomach contents. If no contents are aspirated, inject a bolus of air and listen over epigastrium. Watch for coughing, hoarse speech, cyanosis or dyspnea, any of which might indicate misplacement of the tube into the trachea. If this occurs, remove the tube and attempt reinsertion.

The gastric contents may be aspirated manually or attached to intermittent suction. If continuous suction is all that is available, use a vented NG tube to avoid trauma to the stomach lining.

Occasionally the NG tube might become obstructed or wedged

against the stomach lining, thereby necessitating irrigation or repositioning. Any aspirated contents should be saved for analysis at the hospital.

PROCEDURAL GUIDELINES

1. Select equipment
2. Explain procedure and position patient
3. Measure insertion length from nose to ear to xiphoid and mark with tape
4. Lubricate tube
5. Attach tube to irrigating syringe
6. Slowly and gently insert NG tube through nares as patient swallows
7. Evaluate placement by aspirating for stomach contents; if no contents are aspirated, inject air into the tube and listen over epigastrium with a stethoscope
8. Attach tube to suction, if indicated
9. Tape tube securely in position; avoid pressure on nares; avoid uncomfortable or inconvenient taping
10. Proceed with aspiration or irrigation as directed

NASOTRACHEAL SUCTIONING

Suctioning is removal of obstructive substances from the airway using a catheter attached to a suction source. Suctioning can remove matter by direct aspiration and by stimulating the patient to cough. Respiratory difficulty may occur in a patient who is unconscious, has had a stroke, or is otherwise unable to handle his own secretions. Other conditions which may result in excessive secretions include bronchitis and pulmonary infiltration.

The patient who requires suctioning is usually hypoxic from the obstructed airway before the procedure has begun. This hypoxia is compounded by the use of suction, which draws off available oxygen. To reduce this complication, hyperoxygenate the patient prior to and following the procedure, and keep suctioning intervals as brief as possible.

Deep tracheal suctioning may stimulate the vagus nerve and cause reflex bradycardia. Temporarily discontinue suctioning if this occurs and perform subsequent attempts with caution. Damage to the mucous membrane is another complication. The possibility of this occurring can be reduced by a) avoiding force when passing the catheter, b) lubricating the nasal catheter well, and c) assuring that the suction source is off during insertion of the catheter. Monitor the patient closely during the procedure, give oxygen liberally, and assess the respiratory status regularly to determine the need for further suctioning.

The use of suction can be modified to keep other parts of the airway clear, e.g., clearing the mouth of emesis or blood. When using suction for this purpose, remove the suction catheter and pass the connecting tubing quickly through the mouth and throat. This is usually an emergency maneuver, and is performed without strict regard to technique. Suctioning can also be performed through an endotracheal tube, or nasopharyngeal airway.

PROCEDURAL GUIDELINES

1. Select equipment
2. Inform patient
3. Give patient presuctioning oxygen
4. Position patient in high Fowler's position if conscious; in a supine position if unconscious
5. Connect catheter to suction tubing
6. Lubricate catheter tip with surgical jelly or water
7. Smoothly and steadily insert catheter through nares until reaching carina (patient will cough)
8. Apply suction intermittently, as you rapidly, but smoothly; withdraw catheter, rotating it as it is pulled out
9. Oxygenate patient and allow short rest period
10. Reinsert catheter and repeat process, if needed
11. Suction individual bronchi if necessary by turning patient's head to alternate sides before inserting catheter
12. Observe patient for hypoxia or bradyarrhythmias and delay procedure as indicated
13. Assess and report patient's response to procedure

NEEDLE THORACOSTOMY

Tension pneumothorax is a condition which occurs when air enters the pleural space through a tear in the lung, but is prevented from exiting by a tissue flap that creates a one-way valve effect. The pleural space is inflated with each expiration, subsequently preventing complete lung expansion. If the condition is allowed to persist it can cause collapse of the lung, displacement of the trachea and mediastinum, and eventual bilateral pneumothorax with resultant respiratory collapse.

Signs indicating tension pneumothorax include increasing dyspnea with cyanosis and shock, decreased or absent breath sounds, distended neck veins, and tracheal deviation.

Although tension pneumothorax can be fatal if left untreated, it rarely progresses to a life-threatening stage in less time than it takes to transport the patient. Therefore, it may be more appropriate to transport the patient than to initiate invasive field treatment unless the transport time would be unusually long. If it is determined that the patient is, in fact, suffering from tension pneumothorax and requires immediate relief, a needle thoracostomy may be ordered.

A needle thoracostomy is performed by inserting a large-bore cannula needle into the pleural cavity to reduce the intrathoracic pressure. A rapid rush of air indicates entry into the pleural space. Once this occurs, connect the cannula to a one-way flutter valve and tape it securely in place.

Transport the patient immediately, monitoring vital signs and patient status frequently enroute. Continue ventilatory support with high-flow oxygen and position patient to facilitate air exchange.

In patients with pneumothorax, especially those with tension pneumothorax, who are going to be transported by air, it is imperative that the needle be kept patent. Therefore, these patients should be stabilized in an emergency department prior to air transport, if at all possible.

PROCEDURAL GUIDELINES	1. Identify signs and symptoms indicating a tension pneumothorax
	2. Gather equipment
	3. Properly locate landmarks on the side of pneumothorax: 2nd intercostal space at midclavicular line, or 4th or 5th intercostal space at midclavicular line, or 4th or 5th intercostal space at midaxillary line

4. Prep skin with an antiseptic swab
5. Using aseptic technique, insert cannula at a 90° angle at superior border of rib, approximately 1½ inches into pleural space
6. Listen for rush of air to verify entry into pleural cavity
7. Remove needle and firmly attach flutter valve to cannula
8. Secure cannula and valve to chest wall with tape
9. Transport immediately in position of comfort and continue high-flow oxygen
10. Frequently update vital signs, lung sounds and patient's status
11. Report patient response to procedure

PERICARDIOCENTESIS

Pericardiocentesis is the insertion of a needle into the pericardial sac to remove accumulated blood. It is the treatment of choice for cardiac tamponade, a condition wherein blood accumulates in the pericardial space and quickly suppresses the heart's pumping action. This condition usually results from blunt chest trauma and must be alleviated immediately to prevent circulatory collapse and death.

Cardiac tamponade should be suspected whenever a patient with chest trauma continues to deteriorate despite aggressive therapy. Signs indicating rapid development of tamponade may include muffled or inaudible heart sounds, tachycardia, hypotension, distended neck veins, paradoxical pulse, or signs of profound shock.

When performing a pericardiocentesis, it is important to determine correct landmarks and closely observe the angle of insertion to facilitate entry into the pericardium. Complications that may occur include lacerated coronary artery, ventricular tear, and pneumothorax. Avoid inserting the needle too deeply, as blood might then be aspirated from the ventricle rather than the pericardium. If the first attempt is unsuccessful, repeat the procedure until some fluid can be removed. Normal cardiac output may be restored if even as little as 30 ml can be withdrawn.

Administer high-flow oxygen concurrently, but avoid positive pressure ventilation if possible because it will elevate the intra-thoracic pressure. Monitor and auscultate the chest frequently to assess patient status and determine additional treatment.

PROCEDURAL GUIDELINES

1. Identify indications for procedure
2. Gather and prepare equipment
3. Prepare the patient by applying cardiac monitor, inserting an IV line, and placing patient in a supine position at 60° angle
4. Locate proper injection site, i.e., immediately below left rib cage and slightly to left of xiphoid process
5. Prep skin with antiseptic swab
6. Using aseptic technique, slowly insert the needle 8–10 cm at a 45° angle to the skin; aim toward right sternoclavicular joint; aspirate while inserting
7. Stop inserting needle when blood is aspirated
8. Aspirate available blood, changing syringes if necessary
9. Withdraw needle and apply pressure to puncture site
10. Evaluate patient for improvement in cardiac output and report to base hospital

RADIO COMMUNICATIONS

Communication by mobile radio is a major component of any advanced life support system. It allows the exchange of pertinent information between the scene and the hospital, thereby facilitating management of medical emergencies before arrival at the emergency department.

The key to effective communication with the hospital is the use of an organized format for reporting patient information in clear, concise terms. By giving the hospital a rapid synopsis of the situation, you can help the hospital direct patient care more efficiently. In your initial report give a brief summary of the chief complaint, general patient status, and level of consciousness, as well as an overview of the scene. Avoid diagnosing the patient in your initial transmission, as this may mislead the hospital by limiting the information available to them. Follow this report with an organized summary of the data you have gathered about the patient including age, weight, and sex, a description of the presenting medical problem, pertinent history, physical exam findings, and vital signs. Keep your reports brief and to the point. Use descriptive but appropriate terms,and convey your impressions to the hospital in addition to your actual findings. The specific situation and patient condition may require a varied report format, but always organize your thoughts and communicate them accurately. You might find it helpful to use the field report form as a guide for communicating.

Keep the hospital informed of your actions, particularly if the situation requires pauses in communication. Inform them of changes in patient condition as well as response to treatment. Always speak in a clear voice, maintain a professional manner, and use appropriate medical terms. Repeat all orders for verification, and be courteous and tactful if questions arise. Handle communication difficulties discretely, using alternate communication modes as needed. Avoid unnecessary transmissions, as this will prevent you from assisting your partner and may interrupt the communications of other ALS teams. To prevent confusion among teams, identify your unit and your base hospital with each transmission. In multiple patient incidences, report the most critical patients first, clearly identifying each by assigned number.

PROCEDURAL GUIDELINES

1. Establish communication
   a. turn radio on
   b. select proper channel
   c. call base hospital
   d. identify unit
   e. ask if hospital is copying transmission
2. Use good radio techniques
   a. volume, enunciation, and speed as appropriate
   b. use proper terminology
   c. be concise and express appropriate urgency
3. Give initial report (vary report according to urgency) and include
   a. overview of scene
   b. chief complaint
   c. severity
   d. level of consciousness
4. Report additional patient information
   a. age, sex, weight

b. presenting medical problem
c. pertinent history
d. physical findings
e. vital signs
5. Acknowledge orders from base hospital
   a. repeat exactly as heard and write them down
   b. question unclear orders
   c. provide additional data as requested
6. Report completion of orders and patient response
7. Sign off with final patient report and estimated time of arrival at the hospital

RADIO MECHANICS

Radio mechanics refers to the use of radio hardware to establish two-way communication between the field and the base hospital. Although communication systems vary greatly across the United States, most systems have basic components that are fairly uniform. In most areas of the country, the prehospital provider has three alternatives for field-to-hospital communication: the mobile radio, the telephone, and the ambulance-to-hospital radio. Because of its flexibility, the portable mobile set is usually the first choice. If this frequency is crowded in your area, the telephone might be more appropriate if available. The ambulance-to-hospital frequency is usually reserved as a last resort when other methods are unavailable.

Mobile Radio

All mobile radios used in the United States share the same eight frequencies allocated by the Federal Communications Commission for emergency medical communications. Because these frequencies are limited, the airways are extremely crowded in many high-density areas. In some areas, a central dispatcher selects an available channel for each call, while other areas rely on permanently assigned frequencies for each unit/hospital.

All of these mobile radio frequencies are ultrahigh frequency (UHF) and therefore operate "line-of-sight", i.e., any obstacle between the hospital and the scene (such as a hill or tall building) will interfere with and possibly prevent mobile radio communication.

Sometimes communication can be improved by using a larger antenna or by placing the antenna on a large metal object such as a refrigerator or a metal vehicle. The major drawback to the field radio is the unreliability caused by "deadspot," areas where communication is poor.

To operate the mobile radio, first set the unit as close to the patient as possible. Then turn the unit on, select the appropriate channel and alert the base hospital. In some cases this is done automatically with the first transmission, but in others it is necessary to send a few seconds of EKG calibration in order to alert the hospital that a run is in progress. When speaking, leave the radio in the voice mode, and turn to the calibration or EKG modes only for these purposes. If possible, leave the radio in the "mute" position to avoid broadcasting to all of the people in the room. All mobile radios have knobs for adjusting volume and outside interference. Leave the radio frequency open throughout the run so the hospital can contact you if necessary.

Telephone

If a telephone is available near the patient, the hospital can be dialed through its private line. This is often useful when frequencies are crowded, but is limited because telephones are not always available. Telephone conversations, like field radio conversations, can be recorded at the base hospital for documentation. The telephone can be attached to the radio's telephone coupler to enable the transmission of EKG telemetry to the hospital if desired. Use care in placing a Princess or Trimline style handset into the coupler, as they don't fit snugly and can be easily disconnected.

Ambulance-to-Hospital Radio

The use of this frequency is limited because one member of the team must be in the ambulance. Therefore, it is often faster to transport the patient and contact the hospital enroute. Because these calls do not come through the hospital's base station console, they are not recorded. Since this frequency is not intended for lengthy communication, all calls on this radio should be kept as brief as possible.

If it is not possible to contact the hospital, and your area requires direct contact in order for you to treat the patient, you should limit your care to basic life support and transport the patient immediately.

PROCEDURAL GUIDELINES	**Mobile Radio**

1. Open radio and set up antenna
   a. small gain
   b. high gain (if needed)
   c. augment antenna (if needed)
2. Turn on radio to Voice or "Push to Talk"
3. Adjust volume and/or squelch as needed
4. Send short calibration signal to alert hospital (if needed)
5. Report patient data using an organized format
6. Mute speaker (if requested)
7. Send EKG signal (if requested)

PROCEDURAL GUIDELINES	**Telephone Coupler**

1. Contact hospital over direct land line
2. Attach telephone coupler and communicate through mobile radio over land lines
   a. attach telephone coupler plug into radio
   b. place phone handset into coupler and secure it
   c. turn radio mode to "Telephone"
3. Transmit telemetry over land line via telephone coupler

ROTATING TOURNIQUETS

Rotating tourniquets are constricting bands placed on the extremities of a patient experiencing acute distress from pulmonary edema. They temporarily trap enough blood in the extremities to significantly diminish venous return to the right side of the heart. This procedure helps reduce cardiac workload and lung congestion, thereby alleviating signs of acute distress such as rales, dyspnea and shortness of breath.

Rotating tourniquets are used concurrently with high-flow oxygen, positive-pressure ventilation, and drugs such as morphine sulfate, Lasix, and Aminophylline. Place the tourniquets as high on the extremities as possible to obtain maximum benefit. Do not place a tourniquet on the extremity to which the IV is connected, as that will occlude the flow. Be sure to assess all peripheral pulses after application. Rotate the tourniquets clockwise every 15 minutes and accurately record their placement. Monitor EKG to detect cardiac arrhythmias, and auscultate lungs frequently to assess respiratory changes. If ordered to discontinue this procedure, remove one tourniquet every fifteen minutes. Never remove all tourniquets at once because this will cause sudden engorgement of the heart and lungs, with subsequent deterioration of the patient's condition.

PROCEDURAL GUIDELINES

1. Identify indications for rotating tourniquets
2. Explain procedure to patient
3. Gather equipment
4. Apply tourniquet snugly to:
   a. 3 of 4 extremities, if no IV established
   b. 2 of 3 extremities, if IV established
   c. place tourniquets high on upper arms and thighs
5. Assure that arterial pulses are palpable distal to tourniquets
6. Note time of application and record placement clearly, using stick figures to show positioning of tourniquets
7. Rotate tourniquets clockwise every 15 minutes
   a. apply tourniquet
   b. remove appropriate tourniquet
   c. record timing and rotation pattern accurately
   d. reevaluate pulses
   e. continue pattern of rotation until ordered to discontinue
8. When ordered to terminate procedure, remove one tourniquet every 15 minutes
9. Assess and report patient's response to procedure

VENIPUNCTURE

Venipuncture refers generally to the insertion of a needle into a vein. As used here, venipuncture means drawing a blood sample. In the prehospital setting, a blood sample is necessary to document baseline blood sugar levels prior to administration of glucose to diabetics or unconscious patients.

The primary complication from venipuncture is hematoma formation due to failure to compress the site after the needle has been removed. Avoid unnecessary venipuncture in hemophiliacs or patients on anticoagulants, since excessive bleeding may follow. If an IV line is also being established, a blood sample can be drawn at that time to avoid the need for an additional venipuncture.

Be sure to support the extremity during the procedure. Stabilize the vein to prevent it from rolling. Fill the tubes completely and label each with the proper patient information.

PROCEDURAL GUIDELINES

Venipuncture Using Needle and Syringe

1. Gather equipment
2. Identify an appropriate site (usually antecubital fossa)
3. Apply a constricting band proximal to site and distend vein
4. Prep the skin with antiseptic swab, using a circular motion
5. Insert needle into vein at a 10° angle using aseptic technique, and stabilizing the vein to prevent it from rolling
6. Aspirate to ensure entry and withdraw desired amount of blood
7. Release tourniquet
8. Withdraw needle, applying pressure to the site
9. Inject blood into tube(s)
10. Label tube(s) with patient information
11. Recheck puncture site for bleeding or hematoma
12. Report completion to base hospital

PROCEDURAL GUIDELINES

Venipuncture Using Vacutainer

1. Gather necessary equipment
2. Attach Vacutainer needle to its holder
3. Insert Vacutainer tube into holder (avoid inserting needle into tube and breaking suction)
4. Identify appropriate site (usually antecubital fossa)
5. Apply constricting band proximal to site and distend vein

6. Prep skin with antiseptic swab, using a circular motion
7. Insert needle into vein at a 10° angle using aseptic technique and stabilizing vein to prevent it from rolling
8. Advance tube so needle pierces stopper; check for blood return
9. Allow tube to fill completely; change tubes as needed
10. Release tourniquet
11. Withdraw tube of blood from holder
12. Withdraw needle and apply pressure to site
13. Label tube(s) with patient information
14. Recheck puncture site for bleeding or hematoma
15. Report completion of procedure to base hospital

SELF-ASSESSMENT QUESTIONS

Antishock Trousers

1. Discuss the principles behind the use of the antishock trousers in the management of hemorrhagic shock.

2. List the clinical conditions under which the antishock trousers would be indicated.

3. List the general contraindications for application of the antishock trousers.

4. Describe landmarks for proper placement of the antishock trousers.

5. List sequentially the steps to follow when applying the antishock trousers.

6. How are the antishock trousers applied in the presence of:
   a. impaled objects?
   b. pregnancy/marked abdominal distension?
   c. bowel evisceration?

7. Discuss your actions if the patient complains of increasing respiratory difficulty or nausea and vomiting.

8. When and by whom should the antishock trousers be removed?

9. Describe the complication that will probably result if all three chambers of an antishock suit are suddenly deflated.

Cardioversion

1. List the indications for cardioversion

2. List the accepted w/s settings used in cardioversion of a supraventricular tachycardia for a child and an adult.

3. What is the accepted w/s setting used in cardioversion of ventricular tachycardia?

4. Why is a patient sedated prior to elective cardioversion?

5. What is the drug of choice for sedating a patient prior to cardioversion? Give dosage and route.

6. Define the purpose of synchronization in cardioversion.

7. What is the procedure used in cardioversion?

8. Why must you visualize the blip on the QRS complex and/or the flash of the synchronization button prior to cardioversion?

Carotid Sinus Massage (CSM)

1. What clinical manifestations require the use of vagal stimulation?

2. What are the types of vagal stimulation and in what order are they used?

3. What precautions should be taken prior to vagal stimulation of any kind?

4. Describe the procedure for Valsalva's maneuver.

5. What is the carotid sinus and where is it located?

6. Why is it necessary to check the equality of bilateral carotid pulses prior to CSM?

7. Describe the procedure for carotid sinus massage.

8. When is carotid sinus massage discontinued?

9. Discuss the dangerous side effects which can occur with vagal stimulation.

10. What action(s) should you take if CSM is ineffective?

Chest Auscultation

1. Describe the following lung sounds and discuss the cause and significance of each:
   a. rales
   b. rhonchi
   c. wheezes
   d. decreased breath sounds
   e. absent breath sounds

2. Where are lung sounds best auscultated?

3. What is a pulse deficit and explain its significance?

4. Discuss the implication of muffled heart sounds.

Cricothyrotomy

1. Discuss the indications for cricothyrotomy.

2. Describe the location of the cricothyroid membrane.

3. List the steps followed in performing a cricothyrotomy for the
   a. incision method
   b. puncture method

4. Describe how you would ventilate a patient after a crico-thyrotomy using the following methods.
   a. mouth-to-stoma
   b. ventilator

5. What complications can occur following a cricothyrotomy and how can they be prevented?

6. Describe clinical conditions under which a cricothyrotomy might be required.

Defibrillation

1. Differentiate between defibrillation and cardioversion.

2. What are indications for defibrillation?

3. List the precautions employed while using a defibrillator.

4. Give the formula for calculating the w/s settings used in defibrillation.

5. How do you prepare the paddles for defibrillation?

6. Describe two acceptable sites of paddle placement for defibrillation.

7. List in proper sequence the steps taken prior to defibrillating a patient.

8. What two parameters should be assessed immediately after defibrillation?

9. What drug(s) may be ordered to increase the chances of successful defibrillation?

EKG Monitoring and Telemetry

1. What types of patients would require EKG monitoring?

2. Describe the proper electrode placement for monitoring a patient in the field.

3. List possible causes of artifact and other EKG interference and explain how to trouble-shoot these problems.

4. What skin preparation techniques should be performed to improve the EKG tracing?

5. What would you do if the entire EKG complex was inverted?

6. How do you determine which lead to use to monitor each patient?

7. Why should you avoid unnecessary voice interruptions during the transmission of EKG to the hospital?

8. Why should a calibration signal precede telemetry?

Endotracheal Intubation

1. Discuss the indications for endotracheal intubation.

2. Discuss proper patient positioning and its importance in performing endotracheal intubation.

3. Why is hyperoxygenation important prior to and after the procedure?

4. Describe the procedure of endotracheal intubation.

5. How does one assure proper placement of the endotracheal tube?

6. Discuss the importance of using a bite block (oral airway) with endotracheal intubation.

7. List the complications that can occur during endotracheal intubation.

8. Discuss the importance of cardiac monitoring during endotracheal intubation.

Esophageal Obturator Airway (EOA)

1. When is use of an esophageal obturator airway indicated?

2. List the steps involved in the insertion of an EOA.

3. How much air is used to inflate the cuff of an EOA?

4. Discuss the contraindications for the use of an EOA.

5. What is the proper head and neck position for insertion of an EOA?

6. Discuss the implications of improper placement of the EOA.

7. How do you check for proper placement of the EOA?

8. How do you assess the adequacy of ventilation with the EOA in place?

9. When should an EOA be removed in the field?

10. What phenomenon usually follows removal of an EOA, and what precautions should be taken?

Intracardiac Injections

1. When is an intracardiac (IC) injection indicated in the pre-hospital setting?

2. Name the medications most commonly administered by the intracardiac route, including dosage variances.

3. Give the anatomical landmarks for an IC injection in:
   a. an adult
   b. a child (3–12 years)
   c. an infant (newborn to 3 years)

4. Describe the technique(s) for administration of an IC injection to:
   a. an adult
   b. a child (3–12 years)
   c. an infant (newborn to 3 years)

5. Why is aspiration necessary during advancement of the needle?

6. Why should you inject the medication into the chamber of the heart and not into the muscle?

7. List the potential complications of an IC injection and how they could be prevented.

8. What can you do to assure that CPR is not interrupted any longer than absolutely necessary when you have been ordered to give an IC injection?

9. How would you determine the effectiveness of a medication given by the IC route?

Intramuscular and Subcutaneous Injections

1. When are IM injections given?

2. What sites can be used for IM injections?

3. What is the proper needle size, angle of insertion, and technique for IM injections?

4. List medications that can be given by the IM route.

5. When are SC injections given?

6. What sites can be used for SC injections?

7. What is the proper needle size, angle of insertion, and technique for SC injections?

8. List medications that can be given by the SC route.

9. Why is it necessary to aspirate before injecting any medication?

10. What are possible complications that could arise from IM or SC injections?

IV Insertion Into the External Jugular Vein

1. What are the indications for an external jugular IV in the field?

2. How would you locate the external jugular vein?

3. List in sequence the steps involved in cannulation of the external jugular vein.

4. List the methods for distending the external jugular vein in adults and children.

5. Discuss the possible complications of an external jugular IV and describe how they would present.

6. What should you do if bleeding or infiltration occurs around an external jugular IV?

7. Why would a patient develop a pneumothorax from an external jugular IV? How might you prevent this complication?

IV Insertion Into the Peripheral Vein

1. Discuss the reasons for starting a peripheral IV.

2. What are the various types of needles/cannulas used for an IV and when are they indicated?

3. Describe the criteria used for IV site selection.

4. How do you facilitate venous distension?

5. List the complications of IV therapy and how they appear.

6. How do you keep the vein from rolling during venipuncture?

7. List factors that can alter IV flow rate.

8. What complications can occur if you place tape around the entire extremity in which an IV is running?

IV Insertion Into the Subclavian Vein

1. When is a subclavian IV indicated?

2. What are the landmarks for the subclavian puncture?

3. List in sequence the proper steps in establishing a subclavian IV.

4. What are the possible complications following a subclavian puncture?

5. List three ways to prevent air embolism during subclavian cannulation.

6. What complications can occur if the cannula is moved around after insertion?

IV Medication Administration

1. Why are medications administered intravenously?

2. List field situations in which IV medications may be ordered.

3. List four ways by which medications may be given intravenously.

4. Why is it important to make sure that you are in the vein when injecting a medication?

5. Why must IV drip medications be "piggybacked" into a main IV line?

6. List two things that should be reported to the base hospital following administration of a drug by IV.

IV Set-Up

1. When do you use a pedidrip and why? A maxidrip?

2. When do you use a Volutrol and why?

3. How can you determine that an IV solution is not safe to use?

4. Why would you use extension tubing?

5. Why must the tubing be cleared of air?

6. Discuss the importance of aseptic technique.

7. Discuss factors influencing needle selection.

8. Why is the drip chamber only filled half way?

Magill Forceps

1. Discuss complications which can occur with the use of the laryngoscope.

2. Why is a bite block used in this procedure?

3. When is the use of the Magill forceps indicated?

4. Discuss what precautionary measures are necessary when using the Magill forceps.

5. List in sequence the steps involved in removing an upper airway obstruction with the Magill forceps.

6. What support measures should be utilized during the procedure discussed in question 5?

Nasogastric (NG) Intubation

1. What is the purpose of a nasogastric (NG) tube?

2. When might an NG tube be used in the prehospital setting?

3. How do you measure the length for proper placement of the NG tube?

4. List three methods used to facilitate passage of an NG tube.

5. List in sequence the proper procedure for insertion of an NG tube.

6. List two possible complications from NG tube insertion.

7. If the patient coughs or cannot speak immediately following insertion of an NG tube, what has most likely occurred? What should you do to correct it?

8. How do you confirm proper placement of the NG tube?

9. What does vomiting indicate when an NG tube is in place and attached to suction? How is this corrected?

Nasotracheal Suctioning

1. What is the purpose of nasotracheal suctioning?

2. List several common field situations where suctioning is indicated.

3. How do you position a conscious patient for suctioning? An unconscious patient?

4. List in sequence the proper procedure for nasotracheal suctioning.

5. List two ways to assess that the catheter is in the trachea.

6. Why must high-flow oxygen be given before and after suctioning?

7. Discuss three common complications of nasotracheal suctioning.

8. Describe how to assess the effectiveness of suctioning.

9. Discuss methods of suctioning other than nasotracheal.

Needle Thoracostomy

1. List the signs and symptoms indicating a developing tension pneumothorax.

2. Why is a tension pneumothorax life-threatening?

3. Describe the procedure for relieving a tension pneumothorax.

4. Give two acceptable sites where you may insert the needle to relieve a tension pneumothorax.

5. How do you know when you have entered the pleural cavity?

6. What is the purpose of the flutter valve?

7. What should be included in your patient assessment following needle thoracostomy?

Pericardiocentesis

1. What is the major cause of pericardial tamponade?

2. What are the signs indicating decreased cardiac output and a developing cardiac tamponade?

3. Describe in sequence the steps in performing pericardiocentesis.

4. How can you tell when the needle is in the proper location?

5. What are the complications of pericardiocentesis?

6. What should you do if a puncture is unsuccessful?

Radio Communications

1. What information should be given in the initial radio transmission?

2. Why is it necessary to identify your unit with each transmission?

3. Why is it important to describe the scene?

4. How do you acknowledge a correct drug or treatment order?

5. How do you handle an incorrect drug or treatment order?

Radio Mechanics

1. List three alternative methods for communicating with the hospital and discuss when you would use each.

2. What does "line-of-sight" mean and how does it affect radio communications?

3. How might you augment your antenna?

4. List the steps necessary to communicate over the mobile radio.

5. Discuss the use of
   a. the Mute button
   b. the Squelch button
   c. the Channel Selector
   d. the Radio Mode Selector

6. List the steps necessary to communicate using the telephone coupler.

7. What would you do if you could not establish communications with the hospital?

Rotating Tourniquets

1. Give the indications for use of rotating tourniquets in the field.

2. What are the principles behind the use of rotating tourniquets?

3. How do you apply rotating tourniquets and what precautions should be used?

4. What is the proper system for recording rotation patterns?

5. What complications can occur if all rotating tourniquets are removed at once?

6. List other methods used in the field treatment of pulmonary edema.

Venipuncture

1. When are venipunctures performed in the field?

2. How do you keep a vein from rolling?

3. List three methods that will help distend a vein.

4. List the complications of a venipuncture and how they may be avoided.

5. Describe how you would obtain a blood sample while starting an IV.

BIBLIOGRAPHY

A Paramedic Handbook of Pharmacology. Los Angeles, Los Angeles County Paramedic Program, 1975

Advanced Training Program for Emergency Medical Technician–Ambulance. Prepared for the U.S. Department of Transportation (Contract No. DOT–HS–5–01207) January 1976

American College of Physicians: Endotracheal Intubation. Rocom® Medex International Inc. Production

American Hospital Formulary Service: Hospital Formulary. Washington, DC, American Society of Hospital Pharmacists, 1977

Broedeker EC, Dauber JH: Manual of Medical Therapeutics, 21st ed. Boston, Little, Brown & Co. 1974

Cervenak, Fields, Gravaglia: Principles of Emergency Respiratory Care. Sarasota, Fla, Glen Educational Medical Services

Cole WH, Puestow CB: Emergency Care — Surgical and Medical, 7th ed. New York City, Meredith Corp., 1972

Committee on Trauma, American College of Surgeons: Early Care of the Injured Patient. Philadelphia, WB Saunders, 1972

Condon RE, Nyhus LM: Manual of Surgical Therapeutics, 3rd ed. Boston, Little, Brown & Co, 1976

Dison N: Clinical Nursing Techniques, 3rd ed. St. Louis, CV Mosby, 1975

Dreisbach RH: Handbook of Poisoning. Los Altos, Ca, Lange Medical Publications, 1974

Emergency Product News. GHP Publications, Carlsbad, Ca

Emergency Medicine — Common Emergencies in Daily Practise. Stamford, Conn, Fisher Medical Publications, Inc.

Fuerst EV, Wolff L, Weitzel MH: Fundamentals of Nursing: The Humanities and the Sciences in Nursing, 5th ed. Philadelphia, JB Lippincott, 1974

Gahart BL: Intravenous Medication/Handbook for Nurses and Other Allied Health Personnel. St. Louis, CV Mosby, 1973

Goldman MJ: Principles of Clinical Electrocardiography, 7th ed. Los Altos, Ca, Lange Medical Publications, 1970

Guyton AC: Basic Human Physiology, Normal Function and Mechanisms of Diseases. Philadelphia, WB Saunders, 1971

Huszar RJ: Emergency Cardiac Care. Bowie, Md, Robert J. Brady, 1974

Journal of the American College of Emergency Physicians and the University Association for Emergency Medical Services. St. Louis, CV Mosby

Journal of Emergency Nurses. St. Louis, CV Mosby

Marriott HJ: Practical Electrocardiography, 5th ed. Baltimore, Md, Williams & Wilkins, 1974

Meltzer LE, Dunning AJ: Textbook of Coronary Care. Bowie, Md., The Charles Press, 1972

Meltzer LE, Pinneo R, Kitchell JR: Intensive Coronary Care. A Manual for Nurses. Bowie, Md, Charles Press, 1970

Miller RH, Cantrell JR (eds.): Textbook of Basic Emergency Medicine. St. Louis, CV Mosby, 1975

Paramedics International. La Crescenta, Ca, Paramedics International

Physician's Desk Reference, 29th ed. New Jersey, Medical Economics, 1975

Platt FW: Case Studies in Emergency Medicine. Boston, Little, Brown & Co, 1974

Publishing Sciences Group, Inc: AMA Drug Evaluation, 2nd ed. Littleton, Mass, American Medical Association, 1973

Rose LB, Rose BK: Fundamentals of Mobile Coronary Care. New York City, Medcom Press, 1974

Rakita L, Broder F: Cardiac Arrhythmias Basic Concepts and an Approach to Self-Instruction. Chicago, Year Book Medical Publishers, 1973

Schamroth L: An Introduction to Electrocardiography, 5th ed. Oxford, Blackwell Scientific Publications, 1971

Secor J: Coronary Care, A Nursing Specialty. New York City, Appleton-Century-Crofts, 1971

Sharp L, Rabin B: Nursing in the Coronary Care Unit, 2nd ed. Philadelphia, JB Lippincott, 1970

Shires GT (ed.): Care of the Trauma Patient. New York City, McGraw-Hill, Blakiston Division, 1966

Sproul CW, Mullanney PJ: Emergency Care. St. Louis, CV Mosby, 1974

Standards for Cardiopulmonary Resuscitation and Emergency Cardiac Care. JAMA Supplement, American Medical Association, February, 1974

Stephenson HE Jr. (ed.): Immediate Care of the Acutely Ill and Injured. St. Louis, CV Mosby, 1974

Vinsant MO, Spence MI, Chapell DE: A Common Sense Approach to Coronary Care: A Program. St. Louis, CV Mosby, 1972

Warner CG (ed.): Emergency Care — Assessment and Intervention, 2nd ed., St. Louis, CV Mosby, 1978

Zschoche SA: Mosby's Comprehensive Review of Critical Care. St. Louis, CV Mosby, 1976

INDEX

Index

A

Abdomen, 10
  pain, 11-13, 34, 47, 81-81, 124, 168
  palpation, 9
  trauma, 12, 37, 82-84
Aberrancy, 274
Abnormal behavior, 29, *see also*
  Behavioral emergencies
Abortion
  spontaneous, 46
Absolute refractory period (ARP), 229
Acidosis, 30, 173, 178
Adapin, 188
Adrenaline. *see* Epinephrine
Agonal shock. *see* Low-resistance shock
Aggressive patients, 17, 169
Air embolism, 374, 376, 378
Airway, 5, 36
  management, 14, 31, 48, *see also*
  cricothytotomy; Endotracheal
  intubation obstruction, 13-14,
  51-52, 84-86
Alcohol, 153
  acute intoxication, 16, 41
Aldactazide, 194
Aldactone, 194
Aldomet, 190
Alka Seltzer, 186
Alkalotic agents, 173 ·
Allergic reaction, 86-88, 153, 190, 197
  anaphylactic shock, 15, 33
  asthma, 58
  testing for, 139
Aminophylline, 15, 28, 59, 87, 88, 92,
  93, 107, 130, 137, 149, 163, 192,
  360, 394
Ammonia inhalant, 150
Amnestrogen, 194
Amphetamines, 185
Amphojel, 185
Ampicillin, 187
Amyl nitrate, 186
Analgesics, 97, 167, 184
  contraindications, 13, 32, 41, 82, 83,
  105, 119, 139, 141, 143
Anaphylactic shock, 15, 31, 33, 153,
  155,156,157

Aneurysm, 6, 23, 103-104
  abdominal, 12, 13
Angina, 159, 186
  pectoris, 103, 170
Anhydron, 194
Anorexiants, 184
Antacids, 185
Antianginal agents, 186
Antiarrhythmics, 31, 158, 174, 186, *see*
  also specific drug names
Antibiotics, 186
Anticoagulants, 23, 186
Anticonvulsants, 173, 187
Antidepressants, 188
  tricyclic, 128,171, 188
Antidiarrheal agents, 189
Antiemetic agents, 189
Antihistamines, 153, 190
Antihypertensive agents, 190
Antipsychotic agents, 191
Antishock trousers, 13, 26, 27, 36, 47,
  62, 82, 83, 84, 87, 104, 121, 135,
  141, 143, 355-356
Antispasmodics, 191
Antituberculosis agents, 192
APGAR score, 45, 123
Apnea, 369
Aquatensen, 194
Aquatax, 194
Aramine, 99, 103, 121, 150
  pediatric doses, 100, 122
Arrhythmias, 27, 39, 42, 88-91, 155,
  223-349, *see also* specific type
Aspirin (ASA), 184
Assessment techniques, 5-11
  abdominal pain, 12-13
  multiple patient situations, 37
  multiple trauma patient, 36
  neurological emergencies, 40
  pediatric emergencies, 49-51
  primary survey, 5-6
  secondary survey, 6-11
Asthma, 49, 58, 91-93, 149, 150, 156,
  158, 163, 171, 192
Asystole, 154, 155, 268
Atrial arrhythmias, 193
  fibrillation, 23, 193, 247-249
  flutter, 246-247